The School Nurse's Mental Health Triage Handbook

Evidence-Based Strategies for Assessment, Intervention, and Crisis Response

Patsy Diamond Waller

Table of Contents

Section 1: The 5-Minute Triage – Quick Assessment Tools

Chapter 1.1: Universal Screening Fundamentals

You're standing in your school health office at 7:30 AM, and three students are already waiting outside your door. One looks anxious, another seems withdrawn, and the third appears perfectly fine but mentions having trouble sleeping. How do you quickly figure out who needs immediate attention and who can wait? This is where universal screening becomes your superpower.

Think of universal screening like taking everyone's temperature during flu season. You're not diagnosing the flu, but you're identifying who might need a closer look. Mental health screening works the same way, except instead of checking for fever, you're checking for emotional distress that could interfere with learning, relationships, or safety.

The Evidence Base: Why Screening Matters

Here's something that might surprise you: **early identification of mental health concerns can improve outcomes by up to 70%**. When we catch problems early, before they become full-blown crises, students have a much better chance of getting back on track quickly.

Research consistently shows that students who receive early intervention for mental health concerns demonstrate better academic performance, improved social relationships, and significantly lower rates of serious mental health episodes. But here's the catch – most mental health problems in young people go undetected for months or even years.

Consider this reality: the average time between when a mental health problem first appears and when a young person receives help is **11 years**. That's potentially an entire school career spent struggling silently. Universal screening changes this timeline dramatically.

Studies from major school districts that implemented universal screening programs found several remarkable outcomes. First, they identified three times more students with mental health concerns than traditional referral systems. Second, these students received help an average of 18 months earlier than they would have otherwise. Third, the overall number of mental health crises in schools decreased by 40% within two years.

The National Association of Secondary School Principals found that schools using systematic mental health screening reported fewer disciplinary incidents, improved attendance rates, and higher standardized test scores. When students feel emotionally stable, everything else improves.

But screening isn't just about catching problems – it's about building a culture where mental health matters as much as physical health. When you routinely ask about emotional well-being, you're sending a powerful message that feelings matter and help is available.

Creating Your Screening Schedule: High-Risk Periods

Not all times of the school year are created equal when it comes to mental health challenges. Just like you see more stomach bugs in November and more injuries during PE in September, mental health concerns follow predictable patterns too.

Start of the School Year (August-September)

The beginning of school brings massive transitions, even for students who seem excited to return. New teachers, different schedules, academic pressure, and social reorganization create perfect conditions for anxiety and depression to surface. Plan to complete initial screening within the first month of school, but don't do it during the first week when everyone's still adjusting to basics.

September is also when many students who struggled over the summer finally have access to a caring adult again. You might be the first person to notice that something's not right at home or that a student experienced trauma during the break.

After Extended Breaks (Post-Winter Break, Spring Break)

Long breaks disrupt routines that many students depend on for emotional stability. Students dealing with family conflict, food insecurity, or unsafe home environments often return to school carrying heavy emotional burdens. The contrast between "vacation mode" and academic expectations can trigger anxiety episodes.

Winter break is particularly challenging because it coincides with seasonal depression, holiday stress, and family dynamics. Many students experience their first serious depressive episode during the dark months of December and January.

Following Significant Incidents

Traumatic events – whether they affect one student, a group, or the entire school community – require immediate attention to mental health screening. This includes:

- Deaths of students, staff, or community members
- Natural disasters or community traumas
- School violence or threats
- Serious accidents involving students
- Publicized suicides in the community

After significant incidents, expand your screening to include students who might not obviously be affected. Sometimes the quietest students are processing the most difficult emotions.

High-Stress Academic Periods

Standardized testing seasons, final exams, and college application deadlines create predictable spikes in anxiety and depression. Schedule brief check-ins during these periods, focusing on students who have previously shown signs of academic stress.

Individual Risk Periods

Some students have personal anniversaries that increase their vulnerability – death dates of family members, divorce dates, or trauma anniversaries. Keep a confidential calendar of these dates for students you're monitoring, and plan informal check-ins during these times.

Documentation Requirements: FERPA Compliance

Documentation in mental health screening feels like walking a tightrope. You need enough information to ensure student safety and continuity of care, but you can't violate privacy laws or create records that could harm students later.

What You MUST Document

Document the basic facts of your screening process. Record the date, time, and which screening tool you used. Note the student's responses in objective terms without adding your interpretations. If a student scores above the clinical threshold on a screening tool, document the exact score and what actions you took.

Safety concerns require detailed documentation. If a student reports suicidal thoughts, self-harm behaviors, or mentions being hurt by others, document their exact words as much as possible. Record who you notified and when, what safety measures you put in place, and any follow-up plans.

Document parent contacts related to screening results. Keep records of what information you shared, how parents responded, and what next steps were agreed upon. This protects both you and the family if questions arise later.

What You Should NOT Document

Never document your personal opinions about a student's family situation, appearance, or character. Avoid writing things like "seems depressed" or "probably has anxiety." Stick to observable behaviors and reported symptoms.

Don't document unverified information that students share about others. If a student tells you their friend is using drugs, don't put that in your screening notes. Handle that information according to your school's protocols, but keep it separate from routine screening documentation.

Avoid documenting specific details about trauma or abuse unless you're making a formal report to child protective services. General terms like "reports concerning home situation" are sufficient for screening records.

FERPA-Compliant Record Keeping

Under FERPA, mental health screening records are considered educational records, which means parents have the right to see them (with some exceptions for students over 18 or when safety is a concern). Write your notes with this in mind.

Store screening records separately from academic files when possible. Many schools maintain health records in the nurse's office rather than in cumulative folders. This provides an extra layer of privacy protection.

Remember that FERPA allows sharing of educational records (including mental health screening results) with other school staff who have a "legitimate educational interest." This includes teachers who need to know about accommodations, administrators involved in safety planning, and counselors providing follow-up care.

Retention and Destruction Policies

Most states require keeping mental health screening records for a specific period – usually 3-7 years after the student graduates or transfers. Check your local requirements, but don't keep records longer than necessary.

When you do destroy old records, do it completely. Shred paper documents and permanently delete electronic files. Don't just throw screening forms in the regular trash where they could be found by others.

Parent Communication About Screening

Talking to parents about mental health screening requires finesse. Many parents feel defensive, worried, or skeptical when schools start asking about their child's emotional well-being. Others are relieved that someone finally notices their child might be struggling.

Introducing Screening Programs

Start with education before implementation. Send letters home explaining why mental health screening matters, how it works, and how results will be used. Compare it to vision or hearing screening – routine health checks that help identify students who might need extra support.

Emphasize that screening is not diagnosis. You're not labeling children or putting anything permanent on their records. You're simply checking in on an important aspect of their overall health and development.

Address common concerns directly in your communication. Parents worry that screening will lead to forced medication, removal from their home, or permanent labels. Explain your actual procedures and limitations clearly.

Sample Introduction Script for Parents:

"Good morning, Mrs. Johnson. I'm calling about our universal mental health screening program that we're starting next month. Just like we check students' vision and hearing each year, we're now going to include brief questions about emotional well-being. This helps us identify students who might benefit from extra support before small problems become bigger ones. The screening takes about five minutes and asks questions about things like sleep, anxiety, and mood. If anything concerning comes up, I'll contact you right away to discuss next steps. Do you have any questions about this process?"

Handling Resistance

Some parents will opt their children out of screening, and that's their right. Don't argue or try to convince them. Instead, explain that you're available if concerns arise later, and document their decision.

Other parents might be worried about confidentiality or what happens with the information. Be transparent about your procedures and who will have access to results. Explain that screening results help teachers understand how to better support their child's learning.

Communicating Results

When screening results suggest a student needs further evaluation, approach the conversation as a partnership. You're not delivering a diagnosis – you're sharing observations and offering resources.

"Hi, Mr. Garcia. I wanted to talk with you about Maria's recent health screening. She answered some questions in a way that suggests she might be experiencing more stress than usual. This doesn't mean there's anything wrong with her, but it might be helpful to talk with your family doctor or a counselor about some strategies to help her feel better. I have some resources I can share with you, and I'm happy to help connect you with services if you'd like."

Chapter 1.2: The Essential Assessment Toolkit

Your assessment toolkit is like a well-stocked first aid kit – you need the right tools for different situations, and you need to know how to use them quickly and effectively. But instead of bandages and antiseptic, you're working with questions and conversations that can literally save lives.

The key to successful assessment is having tools that are brief, reliable, and appropriate for school settings. You don't have time for lengthy psychological evaluations, and students don't have patience for complicated questionnaires. You need instruments that give you clear, actionable information in just a few minutes.

ASQ (Ask Suicide-Screening Questions)

The ASQ is your most important tool for identifying students at risk for suicide. Developed by researchers at the National Institute of Mental Health, it's specifically designed for non-mental health professionals working in busy settings. Think of it as the mental health equivalent of checking vital signs.

20-Second Administration Protocol

The beauty of the ASQ is its simplicity. Four questions, asked in order, with clear decision points based on the answers. You can administer it while taking a student's temperature or blood pressure, making it feel like part of routine health care rather than a psychological evaluation.

Here's the exact protocol:

1. "In the past few weeks, have you wished you were dead?"

2. "In the past few weeks, have you felt that you or your family would be better off if you were dead?"

3. "In the past week, have you been having thoughts about killing yourself?"

4. "Have you ever tried to kill yourself?"

If the student answers "yes" to any of these questions, you have a positive screen that requires immediate action. If they answer "no" to all four, you can proceed with confidence that acute suicide risk is low.

Interpretation Flowchart for Ages 8+

The ASQ works for students as young as 8 years old, but you need to adjust your approach based on developmental level. Younger children often need simpler language and more concrete examples.

For elementary students (ages 8-11), try: "Sometimes kids feel so sad or mad that they wish they weren't alive anymore. Have you ever felt like that?" or "Have you ever thought about hurting yourself really badly?"

Middle school students (ages 12-14) usually understand the standard questions but might need reassurance that their answers won't automatically result in their parents being called or them being hospitalized.

High school students (ages 15-18) can typically handle the adult version of the ASQ, but they're often more concerned about confidentiality and what happens next.

Any "yes" answer means immediate action, regardless of age. Don't try to interpret the severity or decide if the student "really means it." A positive ASQ screen means you follow your crisis protocol every single time.

Immediate Response Protocols for Positive Screens

When a student screens positive on the ASQ, your next steps are critical and time-sensitive. First, stay calm and don't overreact.

Students are watching your response to gauge whether they made a mistake by being honest.

Immediately ensure the student is not left alone. If you need to step away or make phone calls, arrange for another trusted adult to stay with them. This isn't just about safety – it's about communicating that you take their feelings seriously.

Next, conduct a brief safety assessment to determine the level of risk. Ask about specific plans, access to means, and protective factors. Questions like "Have you thought about how you would hurt yourself?" and "What has kept you safe so far?" help you understand the urgency of the situation.

Document everything carefully, including the student's exact words when possible. Note the time, who was present, and what immediate safety measures you put in place.

Contact parents or guardians immediately unless doing so would increase risk to the student. In rare cases where family conflict is contributing to suicidal thoughts, you might need to involve child protective services before contacting parents.

Sample Documentation Forms

Your documentation for ASQ screening needs to be thorough but efficient. Create a template that captures essential information without requiring extensive writing during crisis situations.

Include: Student name, date, time, who administered the screening, specific ASQ responses, immediate safety measures taken, parent contact information and response, referrals made, and follow-up plans.

Remember that suicide risk assessments are among the most important documents you'll ever create. They might be reviewed by mental health professionals, attorneys, or administrators, so accuracy and completeness are crucial.

PHQ-9 Modified for Teens

The Patient Health Questionnaire-9 is the gold standard for depression screening in healthcare settings. The teen version maintains the reliability of the original while using language that adolescents understand and relate to.

2-3 Minute Administration Guide

The PHQ-9 asks about nine symptoms of depression over the past two weeks: little interest in activities, feeling down or hopeless, sleep problems, fatigue, appetite changes, feeling bad about yourself, concentration problems, moving slowly or being fidgety, and thoughts of death or self-harm.

Students rate each symptom as "not at all" (0 points), "several days" (1 point), "more than half the days" (2 points), or "nearly every day" (3 points). The total score ranges from 0 to 27, with higher scores indicating more severe depression.

For teens, consider modifying some questions slightly: "Little interest or pleasure in doing things you usually enjoy" instead of just "Little interest or pleasure in doing things." Ask about "feeling tired or having little energy for school or activities" rather than general fatigue.

Scoring Interpretation with Action Thresholds

PHQ-9 scores fall into five categories that guide your response:

- **0-4: Minimal depression** – No immediate action needed, but consider this baseline for future screening

- **5-9: Mild depression** – Monitor closely, consider referral to school counselor, notify parents

- **10-14: Moderate depression** – Definitely refer for counseling, notify parents, consider academic accommodations

- **15-19: Moderately severe depression** – Urgent referral for mental health evaluation, parent meeting required, safety planning

- **20-27: Severe depression** – Immediate mental health evaluation, consider hospitalization, intensive safety planning

These cutoff scores aren't absolute rules – they're guidelines that must be combined with clinical judgment and consideration of other factors like the student's history, current stressors, and support systems.

Question 9 Suicide Risk Protocol

Question 9 of the PHQ-9 asks about "thoughts that you would be better off dead, or thoughts of hurting yourself in some way." This question serves as a suicide screen within the depression assessment.

Any score other than 0 on question 9 triggers your suicide risk protocol, regardless of the total PHQ-9 score. A student could have a low overall depression score but still report suicidal thoughts, which requires immediate attention.

If a student scores 1 on question 9 ("several days"), ask follow-up questions to clarify: "Can you tell me more about those thoughts?" and "Have you thought about how you might hurt yourself?" Document their responses and follow your crisis procedures.

Students who score 2 or 3 on question 9 need immediate safety assessment and likely require emergency mental health evaluation. Don't wait to see if the thoughts pass or assume they're not serious because the student seems to be functioning normally.

Follow-up Scheduling Based on Scores

Your follow-up schedule should match the severity of the student's symptoms:

- **Mild depression (5-9):** Check in within one week, then monthly

- **Moderate depression (10-14)**: Check in within 2-3 days, then weekly

- **Moderately severe depression (15-19)**: Daily check-ins until professional help begins

- **Severe depression (20-27)**: Multiple daily contacts until stabilized with professional care

Keep track of score changes over time. A student whose PHQ-9 score increases from 8 to 14 over a few weeks needs more intensive intervention than someone whose score has remained stable at 14.

GAD-7 for Anxiety

The Generalized Anxiety Disorder-7 questionnaire is your go-to tool for identifying anxiety problems in teens. Like the PHQ-9, it's brief, reliable, and provides clear guidance for next steps.

Age-Appropriate Administration (13+)

The GAD-7 works best for students 13 and older who can understand concepts like "worrying too much" and "being restless." For younger students, you'll need to use behavioral observations and parent/teacher reports rather than self-report questionnaires.

The seven questions ask about anxiety symptoms over the past two weeks: feeling nervous or anxious, not being able to stop worrying, worrying too much about different things, having trouble relaxing, being restless, becoming easily annoyed or irritable, and feeling afraid something awful might happen.

Students rate each item from 0 (not at all) to 3 (nearly every day), giving a total score between 0 and 21.

Cultural Considerations in Interpretation

Anxiety manifests differently across cultures, and your interpretation of GAD-7 results needs to account for these differences. Some cultures view expressing anxiety as weakness or bad luck, leading to underreporting. Others may express anxiety through physical complaints rather than emotional terminology.

Students from cultures that emphasize family honor might be particularly anxious about bringing shame to their families through poor academic performance or behavioral problems. Recent immigrants often experience anxiety related to language barriers, cultural adaptation, and family separation.

Consider involving cultural liaisons or bilingual staff when working with students from different cultural backgrounds. Sometimes anxiety symptoms that seem severe to you are normal responses to very real stressors in the student's life.

Connection to School-Based Interventions

GAD-7 results directly inform the types of school-based support a student might benefit from:

- **Mild anxiety (5-9)**: Relaxation techniques, study skills support, regular check-ins

- **Moderate anxiety (10-14)**: Counseling referral, possible academic accommodations, parent involvement

- **Severe anxiety (15-21)**: Immediate counseling referral, academic modifications, consider medical evaluation

Link anxiety screening results to specific interventions available in your school. If your school has a mindfulness group, students with moderate anxiety might benefit. If you have a quiet space for test-taking, students with severe anxiety might need that accommodation.

Elementary-Specific Tools (Ages 6-11)

Younger students can't reliably complete self-report questionnaires, so your assessment approach needs to be more observational and interactive. Think less "psychological testing" and more "detective work."

Behavioral Observation Checklists

Create checklists that help you systematically observe signs of mental health concerns in younger students. Look for changes in behavior rather than absolute levels – a normally outgoing child who becomes withdrawn is more concerning than a child who has always been quiet.

Key behavioral indicators include:

- Changes in energy levels (suddenly hyperactive or lethargic)

- Appetite changes (not eating lunch, constantly hungry)

- Sleep indicators (falling asleep in class, reporting nightmares)

- Social changes (isolating from friends, clinging to adults)

- Academic changes (sudden drop in performance, inability to concentrate)

- Physical complaints (frequent headaches, stomachaches without medical cause)

- Regression behaviors (baby talk, thumb-sucking in older children)

Document patterns rather than isolated incidents. A child who has three stomachaches in one week might be experiencing anxiety, while one stomachache could be anything.

Non-Verbal Assessment Techniques

Young children often communicate through behavior rather than words. Pay attention to:

- **Play patterns**: Aggressive or repetitive play might indicate trauma or anxiety

- **Art and drawings**: Look for themes of violence, death, or family chaos

- **Body language**: Slumped shoulders, avoiding eye contact, fidgeting

- **Facial expressions**: Flat affect, frequent worried expressions, inappropriate smiling

- **Physical positioning**: Hiding under desks, staying close to exits, avoiding certain areas

Remember that you're looking for patterns and changes, not making diagnoses based on single observations.

Play-Based Assessment Strategies

Use play as a natural way to assess younger children's emotional states. Simple games and activities can reveal concerns that children can't verbalize:

- **Feeling faces**: Ask children to point to faces showing how they feel "today," "at home," or "at school"

- **Family drawings**: Notice who's included, who's missing, and how family members are portrayed

- **Story completion**: Start simple stories and ask children to finish them – their endings often reveal their concerns

- **Puppet play**: Children often say through puppets what they can't say directly

- **Sand tray or toy scenarios**: Watch how children organize play scenes – chaotic arrangements might reflect inner turmoil

Always follow up concerning play themes with gentle questions, but don't over-interpret single instances.

Chapter 1.3: Rapid Triage Decision Trees

When multiple students need your attention simultaneously, you need a system that helps you prioritize quickly and accurately. Your triage system is like air traffic control – making sure the most urgent situations get immediate attention while keeping everyone else safe.

The 3-Level System: Immediate, Urgent, Routine

Immediate (Red Level)

These situations require your attention right now, before anything else. Drop everything and respond immediately:

- Any positive suicide screen or expression of self-harm intent
- Acute psychosis or severely altered mental state
- Panic attacks or severe anxiety episodes
- Aggressive behavior toward self or others
- Disclosure of current abuse or neglect
- Substance use requiring medical attention

Immediate situations get your full attention until they're stabilized or transferred to appropriate care. Don't try to multitask or handle other students while dealing with red-level concerns.

Urgent (Yellow Level)

These students need attention soon – within the same day, preferably within a few hours:

- Moderate depression scores with declining function
- New disclosure of past trauma affecting current behavior

- Significant family crisis affecting the student
- Eating disorder behaviors requiring monitoring
- Social conflicts causing severe distress
- Academic anxiety interfering with performance

Yellow-level students can wait while you handle red-level emergencies, but they shouldn't be forgotten or postponed until the next day.

Routine (Green Level)

These students need follow-up or support, but timing is flexible:

- Mild screening scores with good functioning
- Ongoing monitoring of stable mental health conditions
- Preventive check-ins for high-risk periods
- Academic stress management
- Social skills support
- General wellness concerns

Green-level students can be scheduled for convenient times and don't require immediate disruption of other activities.

Color-Coded Quick Reference Cards

Create physical or digital cards that help you and other staff quickly identify the appropriate triage level. These cards should be simple enough to use in stressful situations but comprehensive enough to cover common scenarios.

Red Card Indicators:

- Student reports wanting to die or hurt themselves
- Student appears confused, disoriented, or out of touch with reality

- Student is hyperventilating, having chest pain, or showing other panic symptoms
- Student is threatening or being violent toward others
- Student reports current abuse, neglect, or exploitation
- Student appears intoxicated or reports taking substances

Yellow Card Indicators:

- Student reports persistent sadness interfering with activities
- Student describes traumatic experiences affecting current functioning
- Student reports family crisis like divorce, death, or major illness
- Student shows signs of eating disorder behaviors
- Student describes peer conflicts causing significant distress
- Student reports academic anxiety affecting sleep or eating

Green Card Indicators:

- Student reports mild worry or stress within normal range
- Student requests someone to talk to about general concerns
- Student shows minor behavior changes noticed by teachers
- Student requests stress management or study skills help
- Student needs follow-up on previously addressed concerns

When to Override Protocol: Clinical Judgment Guidelines

Sometimes your gut tells you something doesn't match the triage guidelines. Trust those instincts – clinical judgment trumps protocols when safety is at stake.

Upgrade Situations (Move to Higher Priority)

Consider moving students to a higher triage level when:

- Multiple risk factors are present even if individual scores are low
- The student's presentation doesn't match their words (saying they're fine but appearing distressed)
- You know additional history that increases risk
- Other staff express significant concerns about the student
- The student's functioning has declined rapidly
- Family or peer relationships are particularly unstable

Downgrade Situations (Move to Lower Priority)

You might move students to lower priority when:

- Strong protective factors are present (supportive family, good coping skills, connected to help)
- The student has effective treatment and support in place
- Symptoms appear related to temporary stressors that are resolving
- The student demonstrates good insight and safety awareness

Never downgrade purely based on time constraints or workload – only when the clinical picture truly supports lower acuity.

Documentation Templates: Triage Decision Documentation Forms

Your triage documentation needs to capture your decision-making process while being quick enough to complete during busy periods.

Essential Elements to Document:

- Date, time, and presenting concern
- Screening tool results (if applicable)

- Triage level assigned and rationale
- Immediate actions taken
- Referrals made or planned
- Follow-up scheduled
- Parent contact (if applicable)

Sample Triage Documentation:

Date: 10/15/24, Time: 10:30 AM Student: Jane Smith, Grade 9 Presenting concern: Teacher referral for withdrawn behavior Assessment: PHQ-9 score 12, denies suicidal ideation Triage level: Yellow (urgent) Actions taken: Parent contacted, counseling referral initiated Follow-up: Check-in scheduled for 10/17/24 Notes: Student cooperative, good insight, supportive family

Keep templates simple and checkbox-friendly when possible. During crisis situations, you need to document quickly without missing important details.

Chapter 1.4: Age-Specific Assessment Modifications

Mental health doesn't look the same at every age. A depressed 7-year-old might complain of stomachaches and cling to their teacher, while a depressed 17-year-old might skip school and isolate from friends. Your assessment approach needs to match the developmental reality of each age group.

Elementary (K-5): Developmental Considerations and Parent Involvement

Elementary students are concrete thinkers who live in the present moment. They can't always identify or articulate their emotions, and they don't yet understand the concept of mental health the way older students do.

Developmental Assessment Modifications:

Young children express distress through behavior and physical symptoms more than words. Instead of asking "Do you feel depressed?" ask "Do you feel sad a lot?" or "Does your tummy hurt when you think about school?"

Use simple language and avoid psychological jargon. Replace "anxiety" with "worried feelings" and "depression" with "sad feelings." Ask about specific situations rather than general emotional states.

Pay attention to developmental regression. A 6-year-old who suddenly starts wetting their pants or a 9-year-old who begins talking in baby talk might be showing signs of emotional distress.

Parent Involvement Protocols:

Elementary students' mental health is closely tied to family functioning, so parent involvement isn't optional – it's essential. Parents often notice changes at home that aren't visible at school, and they're crucial partners in any intervention plan.

Schedule parent meetings for elementary mental health concerns rather than just making phone calls. Face-to-face conversations (even virtual ones) allow you to share observations, answer questions, and develop collaborative plans.

Be prepared to educate parents about childhood mental health. Many parents don't realize that young children can experience anxiety, depression, or trauma symptoms. Provide information about normal vs. concerning behaviors.

Middle School (6-8): Peer Influence Factors and Identity Development

Middle schoolers are navigating the most turbulent developmental period of their lives. Bodies are changing, friendships become intensely important, and identity formation begins in earnest. Mental health concerns often center around peer relationships and self-concept.

Peer Influence Considerations:

Middle school students are extremely sensitive to peer judgment, which affects how they respond to mental health screening. They might minimize problems to avoid seeming different, or they might exaggerate symptoms to gain attention or sympathy.

Assess peer relationships directly. Ask questions like "Who do you sit with at lunch?" and "Who would you call if you had a problem?" Social isolation at this age is a significant risk factor for depression and anxiety.

Pay attention to social media and cyberbullying concerns. Middle schoolers often experience their most intense social conflicts online, and these can have serious mental health impacts.

Identity Development Issues:

Many middle schoolers begin questioning their identity, including sexual orientation and gender identity. These questions are normal but can cause significant distress, especially in unsupportive environments.

Ask open-ended questions about identity concerns: "Are there things about yourself that you're trying to figure out?" rather than making assumptions about specific identity issues.

Be prepared to address body image concerns, which peak during middle school years. Both boys and girls can develop eating disorder symptoms during this period.

High School (9-12): Autonomy Considerations and Substance Use Integration

High school students are transitioning toward adulthood, which affects both their mental health concerns and how you approach assessment. They're dealing with increased academic pressure, relationship complexity, and future planning stress.

Autonomy Considerations:

Older teens want more control over their mental health care and information sharing. Respect their developing autonomy while maintaining appropriate safety oversight.

Discuss confidentiality limits clearly and specifically. High school students need to understand exactly when you'll involve parents or other adults, and they need to feel they have some control over that process.

Allow older teens to be more involved in their own care planning. Ask what kinds of help they think would be useful and what barriers they see to getting support.

Substance Use Screening Integration:

Substance use and mental health problems often occur together in high school students. Integrate substance use questions into your mental health screening rather than treating them as separate issues.

Use non-judgmental language when asking about substance use: "Many teens try alcohol or drugs. Have you used anything that might be affecting how you feel?" rather than "Do you have a drug problem?"

Understand that some substance use might be self-medication for underlying mental health concerns. A student using marijuana daily might be trying to manage anxiety or depression.

Students with Special Needs: Modified Assessment Approaches

Students with developmental disabilities, learning differences, or communication impairments need modified assessment approaches that account for their specific needs and abilities.

Communication Adaptations:

For students with intellectual disabilities, use concrete language and visual supports when possible. Picture cards showing different emotions can be helpful for students who struggle with abstract concepts.

Students with autism might need extra time to process questions and formulate responses. Don't interpret delayed responses as non-cooperation or lack of understanding.

For students with communication impairments, work with speech therapists or special education staff to identify the best way to gather mental health information.

Assessment Modifications:

Some students with special needs might not be able to complete standard screening tools. Rely more heavily on behavioral observations and reports from people who know the student well.

Consider sensory factors that might affect assessment. A student with sensory processing issues might appear anxious when they're actually just overwhelmed by environmental stimuli.

Remember that students with disabilities experience mental health problems at higher rates than their peers, so don't assume that concerning behaviors are "just part of their disability."

Practical Tools for Implementation

Laminated Triage Flowchart

Create a waterproof, durable flowchart that you can keep at your desk or carry with you. Include the key decision points for each triage level and the immediate actions required for each.

Make it visual with color coding and simple symbols. During stressful situations, you need to be able to follow the flowchart quickly without having to read detailed text.

Digital Assessment Forms with Automatic Scoring

If your school uses electronic health records, create digital versions of screening tools that automatically calculate scores and flag concerning responses. This reduces math errors and saves time during busy periods.

Include automatic prompts for follow-up actions based on scores. When a PHQ-9 score reaches the moderate depression range, the system should remind you to schedule parent contact and counseling referral.

Quick-Reference Severity Indicators by Age

Develop age-specific guides that help you quickly identify what's normal versus concerning for different developmental stages. A behavior that's worrying in a 16-year-old might be perfectly normal for a 12-year-old.

Include cultural considerations in your age-specific guides. Some behaviors that seem concerning might be normal expressions of cultural values or family expectations.

Cultural Adaptation Guidelines

Work with your school's cultural liaisons or English language learner staff to understand how mental health symptoms might be expressed differently across cultures. Some cultures express distress through physical symptoms, while others might be more direct about emotional concerns.

Create culturally adapted versions of screening questions when needed, but always maintain the reliability and validity of the original tools.

Understanding that every student brings their own unique combination of developmental stage, cultural background, family dynamics, and individual personality to your health office will make you a more effective screener and a more helpful supporter of student mental health.

Summary: Building Your Foundation for Success

You now have the fundamental tools and knowledge to implement effective mental health screening in your school setting. Universal screening isn't just another task on your already full plate – it's a systematic approach that will actually make your job easier by identifying problems early, before they become crises.

Remember that screening is just the first step. The real impact comes from how you respond to screening results, how you connect students with appropriate resources, and how you build a culture where mental health matters as much as physical health.

Your screening program will evolve over time as you gain experience and learn what works best in your specific school environment. Start with the basic tools outlined here, document what you learn, and adjust your approach based on the needs of your students and community.

The evidence is clear: early identification of mental health concerns saves lives, improves academic outcomes, and creates safer, more supportive school environments. You're not just a school nurse – you're often the first line of defense for student mental health, and these tools give you the confidence and competence to serve in that role effectively.

Section 2: Red Flag Flowcharts

Chapter 2.1: Anxiety Presentations

Sarah walks into your office at 9:15 AM with her hand pressed against her chest, breathing rapidly. "I can't catch my breath," she gasps. "Something's really wrong with me." Her teacher sent her down because she was disrupting math class, but Sarah insists she's having a heart attack. This is the third time this month.

Meanwhile, Marcus hasn't been to PE class in two weeks. His English teacher mentions he's been asking to go to the bathroom frequently during presentations, and the lunch staff says he sits alone every day, picking at his food. Two different students, two different presentations of the same underlying issue: **anxiety**.

Anxiety is probably the most common mental health concern you'll encounter in schools, but it's also one of the most misunderstood. Students, teachers, and even parents often don't recognize anxiety symptoms for what they are. Instead, they see "behavior problems," "attention seeking," or "medical issues." Your job is to cut through the confusion and identify anxiety quickly so you can respond appropriately.

Recognizing Anxiety in School Settings

Anxiety doesn't always look like the stereotypical nervous student biting their nails. In school settings, anxiety wears many disguises, and some of them might surprise you.

Physical Symptoms vs. Psychological Symptoms

The physical symptoms of anxiety often bring students to your office first. These students aren't faking or trying to get out of class – their bodies are genuinely responding to perceived threats, even when those threats aren't physically dangerous.

Common Physical Presentations:

- Rapid heartbeat and chest tightness (often mistaken for cardiac problems)

- Shortness of breath or feeling like they can't get enough air

- Stomach pain, nausea, or digestive issues (the "nervous stomach")

- Headaches, especially tension headaches across the forehead

- Dizziness or feeling lightheaded

- Sweating, trembling, or feeling shaky

- Muscle tension, particularly in shoulders and jaw

- Fatigue from the constant state of alertness

Here's what's happening: when the brain perceives a threat (real or imagined), it activates the sympathetic nervous system. Heart rate increases to pump more blood to muscles. Breathing becomes shallow to take in more oxygen. Digestion slows down because the body doesn't want to waste energy on non-essential functions during an emergency. These are normal, healthy responses – but they're being triggered by things like pop quizzes, social interactions, or presentations rather than actual physical danger.

Psychological Symptoms Often Go Underground:

- Excessive worry about future events (the "what if" thinking spiral)

- Difficulty concentrating or mind going blank

- Irritability or feeling on edge

- Sleep problems (trouble falling asleep, staying asleep, or restless sleep)

- Perfectionism and fear of making mistakes

- Social withdrawal or avoidance of certain activities

- Feeling overwhelmed by normal daily activities

- Constant need for reassurance from adults

Students often hide psychological symptoms because they don't want to seem "crazy" or different from their peers. They might not even recognize these symptoms as anxiety – they just know they feel "off" or "stressed."

Differentiation from Medical Conditions

This is where your nursing skills become crucial. You need to quickly determine when physical symptoms require medical evaluation versus when they're likely anxiety-related.

Red flags that suggest medical evaluation:

- Chest pain with radiation to arm, jaw, or back

- Severe shortness of breath with wheezing or stridor

- High fever accompanying other symptoms

- Abdominal pain with vomiting, especially if severe or persistent

- Headaches with visual changes, confusion, or neurological symptoms

- Any symptom that's completely new for the student or significantly different from their usual pattern

Clues that point toward anxiety:

- Symptoms that come and go, especially in response to specific triggers

- Physical symptoms that improve when the student is distracted or removed from stressful situations

- Multiple vague complaints that don't fit a clear medical pattern

- Symptoms that worsen before tests, presentations, or social events

- Previous episodes with similar symptoms that resolved without medical intervention

Here's a practical approach: **always err on the side of caution for medical symptoms**, but recognize that you can often address both medical and psychological concerns simultaneously. Take vital signs, do a basic assessment, and if everything checks out medically, explore the anxiety angle.

School Avoidance Patterns

Emotionally based school avoidance (EBSA) affects 1-5% of students and represents one of the most serious manifestations of school-based anxiety. This isn't truancy or defiance – it's genuine emotional distress that makes school feel impossible to attend.

Early warning signs of EBSA:

- Increasing requests to call parents or go home

- Frequent visits to your office with physical complaints, especially Monday mornings or after breaks

- Resistance to coming to school after being absent for illness

- Physical symptoms that appear in the morning but resolve once school is dismissed

- Anxiety that peaks on Sunday nights or when preparing for school

EBSA often follows predictable patterns:

Stage 1: Mild resistance – Student complains about school, takes longer to get ready, needs extra encouragement *Stage 2: Physical symptoms emerge* – Headaches, stomachaches, or other complaints appear on school days *Stage 3: Partial avoidance* – Student attends but frequently visits your office, asks to call parents, or leaves early

Stage 4: Complete avoidance – Student refuses to attend or has severe emotional/physical reactions to school

The longer EBSA continues, the harder it becomes to address. Students who miss significant amounts of school fall behind academically, lose social connections, and develop even more anxiety about returning. Early identification and intervention are absolutely critical.

Anxiety Flowchart by Presentation

Different types of anxiety require different immediate responses. Your approach to a student having a panic attack should be very different from your approach to a socially anxious student who's avoiding the cafeteria.

Panic Attacks: 10-Step Intervention Protocol

Panic attacks are intense episodes of fear that peak within minutes. Students experiencing panic attacks often think they're dying, having a heart attack, or "going crazy." Your calm, systematic response can literally be life-changing.

Step 1: Ensure immediate safety – Move the student to a quiet, private space if possible. Remove them from audiences or chaotic environments.

Step 2: Introduce yourself and stay calm – "Hi, I'm Mrs. Johnson, the school nurse. I'm here to help you. You're safe."

Step 3: Validate their experience – "This feels really scary right now, but you're not in physical danger."

Step 4: Check vital signs quickly – Take pulse and blood pressure if possible, but don't make this feel like a medical emergency unless it truly is one.

Step 5: Guide their breathing – "We're going to slow your breathing down. Breathe in slowly through your nose for 4 counts... hold for 4... out through your mouth for 6."

Step 6: Use grounding techniques – Help them identify 5 things they can see, 4 things they can touch, 3 things they can hear, 2 things they can smell, 1 thing they can taste.

Step 7: Provide reassurance about duration – "Panic attacks feel terrible, but they peak in about 10 minutes and then start to get better."

Step 8: Stay with them through the episode – Don't leave them alone, even if other students need attention.

Step 9: Debrief when they're calmer – "What was happening right before this started?" Help them identify triggers.

Step 10: Plan next steps – Contact parents, schedule follow-up, consider referral for ongoing support.

Social Anxiety: Classroom Accommodation Recommendations

Students with social anxiety often fly under the radar because they're quiet and compliant. They're not disruptive, so teachers might not realize they're struggling significantly.

Immediate accommodations you can suggest:

- Allow extra time to respond to questions (don't call on them unexpectedly)
- Permit alternative ways to demonstrate knowledge (written responses instead of oral presentations)
- Provide advance notice about presentations or group work
- Allow them to sit near the door or in a less prominent location
- Give options for participation (writing on the board vs. speaking aloud)
- Create opportunities for one-on-one interaction with teachers

Longer-term strategies:

- Gradual exposure to social situations with support

36

- Social skills groups or peer mentoring programs

- Connection with other socially anxious students who can support each other

- Family education about social anxiety and home support strategies

Generalized Anxiety: Progressive Intervention Ladder

Students with generalized anxiety worry about everything – academics, family, health, the future, things that happened in the past. Their anxiety isn't specific to one situation, so your intervention needs to be more comprehensive.

Level 1 - Basic support:

- Regular check-ins to monitor anxiety levels

- Teach basic relaxation techniques (deep breathing, progressive muscle relaxation)

- Help identify and challenge unrealistic worry thoughts

- Connect with school counselor for ongoing support

Level 2 - Increased intensity:

- More frequent check-ins (daily or multiple times per day)

- Specific coping strategies for high-anxiety periods

- Possible academic accommodations (extended time, quiet testing space)

- Parent involvement and home-school communication

Level 3 - Intensive intervention:

- Consider external mental health referral

- Possible medication evaluation

- Significant academic modifications

- Crisis planning for severe anxiety episodes

Test Anxiety: Immediate and Long-term Strategies

Test anxiety is incredibly common and can seriously impact academic performance, creating a cycle where poor performance increases anxiety, which leads to worse performance.

Immediate strategies for test day:

- Allow extra time when possible
- Provide a quiet, less distracting environment
- Permit breaks during lengthy exams
- Allow students to use relaxation techniques during tests
- Consider alternative assessment formats when appropriate

Long-term strategies:

- Teach test-taking strategies and study skills
- Practice relaxation techniques regularly, not just during tests
- Address perfectionist thinking patterns
- Build confidence through smaller, low-stakes assessments
- Work with teachers to modify testing approaches when needed

De-escalation Techniques

When a student is in the midst of an anxiety episode, your first goal is to help them regain control of their nervous system. These techniques work because they activate the parasympathetic nervous system (the "rest and digest" response) which counteracts the fight-or-flight response driving their anxiety.

5-4-3-2-1 Grounding Technique

This technique works by redirecting attention away from internal anxiety symptoms toward external, concrete sensory information. It's particularly effective because it's simple to remember and can be done anywhere.

"Let's try something together. Look around and tell me 5 things you can see... Good. Now 4 things you can physically touch... Now 3 things you can hear... 2 things you can smell... and 1 thing you can taste."

The key is to make this interactive, not just a set of instructions. Ask follow-up questions: "What does that desk feel like when you touch it?" or "Tell me more about that sound you're hearing." This keeps their attention focused outward instead of on their anxiety symptoms.

Modify for different ages:

- Elementary students might need more guidance: "I see a red poster on the wall – what else do you see that's red?"

- Middle schoolers often respond well to making it a game: "Can you find something blue, something soft, something that makes noise?"

- High schoolers usually prefer straightforward instructions but appreciate knowing why it works

Box Breathing Instruction Cards

Box breathing (also called square breathing) is one of the most effective techniques for activating the parasympathetic nervous system. The specific pattern of equal counts for inhaling, holding, exhaling, and holding creates a rhythm that naturally calms the nervous system.

Basic box breathing pattern:

- Breathe in for 4 counts

- Hold for 4 counts

- Breathe out for 6 counts

- Hold for 4 counts

- Repeat 4-6 times

Create visual instruction cards that students can keep with them. Include simple drawings of a square with arrows showing the breathing pattern, and use colors (blue for breathing in, red for breathing out).

Modifications for different situations:

- Younger students might need shorter counts (3-3-4-3)

- Students in crisis might start with natural breathing and gradually move to counted breathing

- Some students respond better to 4-7-8 breathing (in for 4, hold for 7, out for 8)

Teaching tips:

- Model the breathing yourself first

- Use your hand to show the rhythm

- Don't worry if they don't get it perfect – any controlled breathing helps

- Practice when they're calm, not just during anxiety episodes

Safe Space Creation in Nursing Office

Your office can become a sanctuary for anxious students, but this requires intentional design and clear boundaries.

Physical environment considerations:

- Keep lighting soft rather than harsh fluorescent when possible

- Have comfortable seating options (not just medical exam chairs)

- Include calming visual elements (nature photos, soft colors)

- Minimize clutter and overstimulating decorations
- Ensure privacy – students need to feel safe from observation by peers

Sensory tools to keep available:

- Stress balls or fidget toys for tactile grounding
- Soft blankets for comfort
- Essential oils or calming scents (if school policy allows)
- Quiet background music or white noise options
- Hot/cold packs for physical comfort

Establish clear protocols:

- Students know they can come to you when feeling overwhelmed
- Set time limits to prevent avoidance of all school activities
- Create signals students can use to request help without disrupting class
- Train other staff about when to send students to you vs. handling anxiety in the classroom

Return-to-Class Protocols

Getting students back to class after an anxiety episode requires careful timing and preparation. Send them back too soon, and the anxiety might return immediately. Wait too long, and you're reinforcing avoidance patterns.

Readiness Assessment Checklist

Before sending a student back to class, check these indicators:

Physical signs of readiness:

- Breathing has returned to normal rhythm

41

- Heart rate has decreased (you can check pulse or simply observe)

- Muscle tension has decreased (shoulders relaxed, hands unclenched)

- Color has returned to normal (less pale or flushed)

Emotional signs of readiness:

- Student can talk about what happened without becoming re-anxious

- They express willingness to return to class

- They can identify what might help if anxiety returns

- They seem grounded and present rather than "spacey" or disconnected

Cognitive signs of readiness:

- Can focus on conversation without being distracted by anxiety

- Can problem-solve about returning to class

- Remembers and can use coping strategies you practiced together

Don't rush this process. An extra 10 minutes in your office is better than having the student return to class only to need to come back 20 minutes later.

Teacher Communication Templates

Teachers need to know how to support students returning from anxiety episodes, but they also need clear, brief information that respects student privacy.

Basic return-to-class communication: "Sarah is returning to class. She's feeling better but might need a few minutes to get settled back in. Please check in with her quietly in about 15 minutes to see how she's doing."

For students with ongoing anxiety issues: "Marcus is working on managing some stress right now. He might need occasional breaks or a chance to step into the hallway if he's feeling overwhelmed. Please send him back to me if he asks, and let me know if you notice signs that he's struggling."

For teachers who need more specific guidance: "Emma sometimes experiences physical symptoms when she's anxious – she might put her head down, ask to get water, or seem distracted. These are signs she's trying to cope, not being defiant. If you see these signs, you can quietly ask if she needs to visit me."

Follow-up Scheduling

Consistent follow-up is what separates effective anxiety intervention from just crisis management. Students need to know that someone is paying attention to their mental health over time, not just during acute episodes.

Same-day follow-up:

- Check in before dismissal to see how the rest of the day went
- Ask what worked well and what was still challenging
- Make sure they have a plan for managing evening anxiety (homework worries, social media anxiety)

Next-day follow-up:

- Brief morning check-in: "How was your evening? How are you feeling about today?"
- Touch base with teachers about how the student did in class
- Adjust support plans based on what you learned from the previous day

Weekly follow-up for ongoing anxiety:

- Track patterns: what days/times/situations are most challenging?

- Review and practice coping strategies regularly

- Monitor for improvements or worsening symptoms

- Communicate with parents about what you're seeing at school

Monthly follow-up for stable students:

- Celebrate progress and improvements

- Update coping strategy "toolkit" with new techniques

- Assess whether current level of support is still appropriate

- Plan for upcoming stressful periods (testing season, transitions)

Chapter 2.2: Depression Indicators

Depression in children and teens often looks nothing like depression in adults. While adults might withdraw to their bedrooms and sleep all day, a depressed 8-year-old might complain of stomachaches every morning. A depressed 16-year-old might start getting into fights or experimenting with drugs. Your challenge is recognizing depression across all its developmental disguises.

Think of depression as an internal storm system. Sometimes it's obvious – dark clouds, heavy rain, thunder that everyone can hear. But sometimes it's more subtle – a gradual dimming of light, a persistent chill, a heaviness in the air that's hard to name. Students experiencing depression might not even realize that's what's happening to them. They just know they don't feel right.

Early Warning Signs by Age Group

Depression symptoms change dramatically across developmental stages, partly because children and teens have different cognitive and emotional capacities, and partly because depression interacts with the typical challenges of each age group.

Elementary: Somatic Complaints and Regression Behaviors

Young children don't have the emotional vocabulary to say "I feel depressed." Instead, their bodies and behaviors do the talking. Elementary school depression often masquerades as physical problems or behavioral regression.

Physical complaints that may signal depression:

- Frequent headaches or stomachaches, especially on school days

- Changes in appetite (eating much more or much less than usual)

- Sleep problems (difficulty falling asleep, nightmares, or sleeping much more than typical)

- Fatigue or low energy that isn't explained by illness or poor sleep

- Frequent minor injuries or complaints that seem disproportionate to the actual problem

Behavioral regression signals:

- Previously potty-trained children having accidents

- Thumb sucking, baby talk, or other infantile behaviors in older children

- Increased clinginess to parents or teachers

- Separation anxiety that seems excessive for the child's age

- Loss of previously mastered skills (academic or social)

Other elementary depression indicators:

- Withdrawal from activities they previously enjoyed

- Play themes that focus on death, sadness, or abandonment

- Increased irritability or emotional outbursts over minor issues

- Difficulty concentrating or completing tasks they could do before

- Social isolation or rejection by peers

Here's what's happening developmentally: Young children are concrete thinkers who experience emotions in their bodies. They don't understand concepts like "feeling hopeless" but they do understand "my tummy hurts" or "I want my mommy." Regression behaviors are often attempts to return to a time when they felt safer and more cared for.

Middle School: Social Withdrawal and Academic Decline

Middle schoolers are developmentally focused on peer relationships and beginning to form their identity. Depression at this age often shows up through disruptions in these key developmental tasks.

Social withdrawal patterns:

- Eating lunch alone or not eating lunch at all
- Dropping out of activities, sports, or clubs they previously enjoyed
- Not participating in classroom discussions or group work
- Avoiding social media or becoming obsessed with it
- Reporting that friends are "stupid" or "annoying" when previously they were important
- Spending more time with adults than peers

Academic decline indicators:

- Grades dropping in multiple subjects (not just one difficult class)
- Missing assignments or turning in incomplete work
- Teachers reporting the student seems "disconnected" or "not present"
- Difficulty concentrating during class
- No longer asking questions or seeking help when confused

Middle school specific signs:

- Extreme sensitivity to criticism or perceived rejection

- Black-and-white thinking ("everyone hates me," "I'm the worst student")

- Increased conflicts with parents or authority figures

- Experimentation with different identities or dramatic personality changes

- Physical complaints that interfere with participation in activities

The middle school years are when many students first experience serious depression because this is when abstract thinking develops. Suddenly, they can contemplate concepts like "forever," "never," and "hopeless" in ways they couldn't before. This cognitive development, combined with hormonal changes and social pressures, creates perfect conditions for depression to emerge.

High School: Substance Use and Risky Behaviors

Teenagers have more freedom and access to potentially harmful behaviors, so depression in high school often manifests through dangerous choices rather than just withdrawal or academic problems.

Substance use red flags:

- Coming to school smelling like alcohol or marijuana

- Dramatic personality changes that might indicate regular substance use

- New friend groups associated with substance use

- Missing school on Mondays or after weekends (potential hangover recovery)

- Academic performance that fluctuates wildly

Risky behavior indicators:

- Reckless driving or getting into accidents

- Sexual behavior that's impulsive or dangerous

- Self-injury behaviors (cutting, burning, hitting themselves)

- Getting into physical fights or legal trouble

- Dramatic changes in appearance or personal hygiene

High school depression also includes:

- Sleep schedule disruptions (staying up very late, sleeping through alarms)

- Loss of interest in future planning (college applications, career thinking)

- Cynical or hopeless talk about the world, relationships, or their future

- Social media posts that hint at depression or self-harm

- Dropping advanced classes or reducing course load significantly

Adolescent depression is particularly dangerous because teens have adult-level access to potentially lethal means (cars, substances, weapons) but don't yet have fully developed judgment and impulse control. The combination of intense emotional pain and poor decision-making capacity can be deadly.

Depression Severity Assessment

Not all depression looks the same, and your response needs to match the severity of what you're seeing. A mildly depressed student might need counseling and extra support, while a severely depressed student might need immediate safety planning and emergency intervention.

PHQ-9 Interpretation with School-Specific Actions

The PHQ-9 gives you a standardized way to measure depression severity, but you need to know how to translate those scores into concrete actions within your school setting.

Minimal Depression (PHQ-9: 0-4)

- *What this looks like:* Student reports occasional sadness or low mood but is generally functioning well

- *School actions:* Document baseline score, provide general mental health resources, schedule routine follow-up in 2-4 weeks

- *Teacher communication:* No special accommodations needed, but let teachers know you're monitoring

- *Parent involvement:* Inform parents of screening results, provide prevention resources

Mild Depression (PHQ-9: 5-9)

- *What this looks like:* Student reports some depression symptoms that are beginning to interfere with daily activities

- *School actions:* Weekly check-ins, connect with school counselor, provide coping strategy resources

- *Teacher communication:* Request teachers watch for changes in academic performance or social engagement

- *Parent involvement:* Meeting to discuss findings, provide community mental health resources, develop home-school communication plan

Moderate Depression (PHQ-9: 10-14)

- *What this looks like:* Student reports multiple depression symptoms that significantly impact functioning

- *School actions:* Twice-weekly check-ins, formal counseling referral, consider academic accommodations

- *Teacher communication:* Specific accommodation requests (extended deadlines, alternative assignments)

- *Parent involvement:* Urgent meeting to discuss professional mental health evaluation, coordinate care plan

Moderately Severe Depression (PHQ-9: 15-19)

- *What this looks like:* Student reports severe depression symptoms that make normal functioning very difficult

- *School actions:* Daily check-ins, immediate professional referral, academic modifications, safety planning

- *Teacher communication:* Significant accommodations needed, possible modified schedule

- *Parent involvement:* Same-day contact, strong recommendation for immediate professional evaluation

Severe Depression (PHQ-9: 20-27)

- *What this looks like:* Student reports pervasive depression symptoms that make functioning extremely difficult

- *School actions:* Multiple daily check-ins, emergency mental health referral, comprehensive safety planning, consider homebound instruction

- *Teacher communication:* Major modifications or temporary withdrawal from regular classes

- *Parent involvement:* Immediate contact, possible recommendation for hospitalization or intensive treatment

Functional Impairment Evaluation

PHQ-9 scores tell you about symptom severity, but functional impairment tells you about real-world impact. A student might have a moderate PHQ-9 score but if their depression is preventing them from attending school or maintaining relationships, the functional impairment is severe.

Academic function assessment:

- Are they completing assignments at their usual level?
- Has their participation in class changed?
- Are they able to concentrate during instruction?
- Are they asking for help when needed?
- How does their current performance compare to previous terms?

Social function assessment:

- Are they maintaining friendships?
- Do they participate in lunch, recess, or social activities?
- Are they engaging with family members normally?
- Have they withdrawn from activities they previously enjoyed?
- Are they able to communicate their needs appropriately?

Daily living function assessment:

- Are they maintaining personal hygiene?
- Are they sleeping and eating regularly?
- Can they get themselves ready for school independently?
- Are they able to handle normal daily stressors?
- Do they have energy for basic self-care tasks?

Parent Notification Decision Tree

Deciding when and how to involve parents in depression concerns requires balancing student autonomy, safety needs, and legal requirements.

Always notify parents immediately:

- Any suicide risk or self-harm behaviors

- Severe depression that significantly impairs functioning

- Substance use in conjunction with depression symptoms

- Any situation where safety is a concern

Notify parents within 24-48 hours:

- Moderate depression that affects academic performance

- Depression symptoms that represent a significant change from baseline

- When professional evaluation is recommended

- When academic accommodations are needed

Consider student input before notifying parents:

- Mild depression in older teens with good insight

- When family conflict might be contributing to depression

- For students who have demonstrated good judgment and safety awareness

Don't notify parents (rare exceptions):

- When doing so would increase risk to the student

- When abuse or neglect by parents is suspected

- When legal consultation suggests waiting (very unusual)

Immediate Interventions

When you identify depression in a student, your immediate response can set the tone for their entire recovery process. Students are watching to see if you take their feelings seriously, if you have confidence in helping them, and if you can provide hope that things can get better.

Safety Assessment Protocol

Every student with depression needs at least a basic safety assessment, even if they don't report suicidal thoughts. Depression and suicide risk are closely linked, and you need to know where each student stands.

Basic safety questions:

- "Sometimes when people feel this sad, they have thoughts about not wanting to be alive. Have you had thoughts like that?"

- "Have you ever thought about hurting yourself in any way?"

- "What helps you feel better when you're having a really hard time?"

- "Who are the people you can talk to when you're struggling?"

- "What are some reasons you have to keep going, even when things are difficult?"

If they report any safety concerns:

- Use the ASQ (Ask Suicide-Screening Questions) protocol immediately

- Don't leave them alone

- Contact parents and mental health professionals

- Develop immediate safety planning

- Document everything thoroughly

If safety assessment is reassuring:

- Explore their existing coping strategies

- Help them identify supportive people in their life

- Discuss what typically helps when they're feeling down

- Plan regular check-ins to monitor safety over time

Supportive Communication Scripts

How you talk to depressed students matters enormously. Your words can provide hope and connection, or they can inadvertently make students feel more isolated and misunderstood.

Validation scripts:

- "It sounds like you're going through a really difficult time right now."

- "Thank you for trusting me enough to tell me how you're feeling."

- "Depression can make everything feel much harder than it normally would."

- "You're not alone in feeling this way, and there are people who want to help you."

Hope-instilling scripts:

- "Depression is treatable. Many people feel much better with the right help."

- "You've gotten through hard times before, and we can figure out how to get through this too."

- "Even though it doesn't feel like it right now, these feelings can change."

- "Let's work together to find some ways to help you feel better."

Avoid these phrases:

- "Just think positive" or "Look on the bright side"

- "Everyone feels sad sometimes" (minimizes their experience)

- "You have so much to be grateful for" (creates guilt)

- "Snap out of it" or "You just need to try harder"

- "This is just a phase" (dismisses their pain)

Connection to School Counselor Protocols

School counselors are your key partners in supporting depressed students, but the referral process needs to be handled thoughtfully to ensure students follow through and benefit from counseling services.

Making effective referrals:

- Prepare students for what to expect from counseling
- Provide specific information about why you think counseling would help
- Address concerns or resistance they might have
- Schedule the first appointment while they're with you when possible
- Offer to walk them to their first appointment if they're anxious

Information to provide to counselors:

- Specific depression symptoms and severity
- Functional impairment you've observed
- Safety assessment results
- Family dynamics or stressors you're aware of
- Student's strengths and existing coping strategies
- Any accommodations or supports that seem helpful

Monitoring Systems

Depression isn't a crisis that gets resolved in a day or week. It's an ongoing condition that requires systematic monitoring to track progress, identify setbacks early, and adjust interventions as needed.

Daily Check-in Procedures

For students with moderate to severe depression, daily contact helps prevent small setbacks from becoming major crises. But daily check-ins need to be brief and sustainable, or they'll become burdensome for both you and the student.

Structured daily check-in format:

- *Mood check:* "On a scale of 1-10, how has your mood been today?"

- *Function check:* "How did you do with school stuff today?"

- *Social check:* "How were things with friends/family today?"

- *Coping check:* "Did you use any of the strategies we talked about?"

- *Tomorrow planning:* "What's one thing you're looking forward to tomorrow?"

Keep a simple log of these check-ins. Patterns often emerge that aren't obvious from individual conversations – maybe Mondays are consistently harder, or mood dips every few weeks in a predictable cycle.

Academic Performance Tracking

Depression significantly impacts academic performance, and academic struggles can worsen depression. Breaking this cycle requires systematic attention to how students are doing in their classes.

Weekly academic monitoring:

- Check grades in online systems if available

- Touch base with core teachers about assignment completion

- Monitor attendance patterns in different classes

- Track requests for extensions or accommodations

- Note any classes where performance is particularly affected

Work with teachers to identify:

- Assignments that seem overwhelming or impossible for the depressed student

- Times of day when the student functions better or worse

- Subjects where depression impact is most severe

- Classroom modifications that seem to help

- Signs that depression is improving or worsening

Attendance Pattern Analysis

Attendance patterns often reveal depression patterns that aren't obvious from conversations with students. Depressed students might not realize they're missing school more often or that their absences follow predictable patterns.

Track these attendance indicators:

- Days of the week most often missed (Monday absences suggest weekend depression)

- Partial day patterns (leaving early, arriving late, missing specific classes)

- Absences around stressful events (tests, presentations, social events)

- Medical excuse patterns (frequent headaches, stomachaches on school days)

- Seasonal patterns (increased absences during darker months)

Use attendance data to:

- Identify triggers that make school avoidance more likely

- Plan extra support during high-risk periods

- Modify schedules or expectations during difficult times

- Celebrate improvements in attendance as signs of recovery

- Alert parents and teachers when concerning patterns emerge

Depression recovery isn't linear – students have good days and bad days, good weeks and difficult weeks. Your monitoring systems help you see the overall trajectory while responding appropriately to daily fluctuations. Most importantly, they demonstrate to students that their mental health matters and that they're not going through this alone.

Chapter 2.3: Self-Harm Behaviors

The first time you discover that a student has been cutting themselves, your heart might skip a beat. The neat rows of healing cuts on their arm, the fresh scratches hidden under long sleeves, the concerning doodles in their notebook margins – these discoveries can shake even experienced school nurses.

Self-harm behaviors are more common than many people realize, with studies suggesting that 15-20% of teens engage in some form of self-injury. But these behaviors are also deeply misunderstood. Students who self-harm aren't necessarily suicidal, though they are at higher risk. They're not seeking attention, though they do need attention. They're using physical pain to manage emotional pain that feels unbearable.

Your response to discovering self-harm can literally change a student's trajectory. Handle it with skill and compassion, and you might be the turning point that helps them find healthier coping strategies. Handle it poorly, and you might drive the behavior underground where it becomes more dangerous and harder to address.

Identification and Initial Response

Self-harm behaviors exist on a spectrum from relatively minor tissue damage to serious injuries that require medical attention. Your job is to quickly assess both the physical and emotional components of what you're seeing.

Types of Self-Harm Behaviors

Cutting is the most common and recognizable form of self-harm, but it's far from the only method students use:

- *Cutting with razor blades, knives, scissors, or other sharp objects* – usually on arms, legs, or torso

- *Burning with cigarettes, matches, hot objects, or chemicals* – often on hands, arms, or areas hidden by clothing

- *Hitting or punching themselves or objects* – walls, lockers, trees, leading to bruised knuckles or other injuries

- *Scratching or picking* at skin, wounds, or scabs until they cause significant damage

- *Hair pulling* (trichotillomania) that creates bald patches or thin spots

- *Interference with wound healing* by picking at cuts or burns to keep them from healing properly

- *Carving words or symbols* into skin, often with emotional significance

- *Head banging* or other forms of blunt force trauma

Students often progress from less severe methods to more severe ones over time, or they might use different methods depending on their emotional state or available privacy.

Immediate Medical Assessment

When you discover self-harm, your first priority is always the physical safety of the student. Some self-inflicted injuries require immediate medical attention, while others can be treated with basic first aid.

Injuries requiring emergency medical care:

- Deep cuts that expose fat, muscle, or bone

- Any cut longer than 1-2 inches or gaping open

- Burns covering significant surface area or showing signs of infection

- Injuries to face, neck, genitals, or joints

- Any injury that won't stop bleeding with direct pressure
- Signs of infection: red streaks, pus, fever, excessive swelling

Injuries you can manage in your office:

- Superficial cuts that have stopped bleeding
- Small burns without signs of infection
- Bruises or minor tissue damage from hitting
- Scratches or picking wounds that aren't actively bleeding

Basic wound care for self-harm injuries:

- Clean your hands and use universal precautions
- Clean the wound gently with saline or clean water
- Apply antibiotic ointment if available and not contraindicated
- Cover with appropriate bandaging
- Document the injury location, size, and appearance
- Provide the student with clean bandages for ongoing care

Safety Planning in School Setting

Once you've addressed immediate medical needs, you need to assess ongoing safety and develop a plan to keep the student safe while at school.

Immediate safety questions:

- "Are you thinking about hurting yourself again today?"
- "Do you have anything with you that you might use to hurt yourself?"
- "What usually happens right before you hurt yourself?"
- "What helps you when you're feeling the urge to hurt yourself?"

School-based safety planning:

- Identify safe adults the student can approach when feeling urges to self-harm

- Create a plan for storing or removing potential instruments (scissors, compasses, etc.)

- Establish check-in times throughout the school day

- Identify safe spaces where the student can go when feeling overwhelmed

- Teach alternative coping strategies for managing difficult emotions

Environmental modifications:

- Consider bathroom monitoring if that's where self-harm is occurring

- Work with teachers to be aware of potential instruments in their classrooms

- Create a signal system for the student to request help without embarrassment

- Ensure the student is never left unsupervised when safety risk is high

Risk Assessment Protocols

Self-harm and suicide risk are related but distinct issues. Many students who self-harm are not trying to kill themselves – they're trying to feel better, to feel something, or to express emotions they can't put into words. However, self-harm does increase suicide risk, so careful assessment is essential.

Columbia Suicide Severity Rating Scale Adaptation

The C-SSRS can be adapted for use with students who self-harm to help you distinguish between non-suicidal self-injury and potentially suicidal behaviors.

Key questions to differentiate intent:

- "When you hurt yourself, are you trying to end your life or are you trying to feel better?"

- "Have you ever hurt yourself in a way that you thought might kill you?"

- "Have you ever hurt yourself and hoped that you might die from it?"

- "Do you think about dying when you're hurting yourself?"

Risk levels based on C-SSRS adaptation:

Low risk: Student reports self-harm for emotional relief, denies suicidal intent, has good safety awareness, identifies reasons for living

Moderate risk: Student reports occasional thoughts about death while self-harming, some ambivalence about living, self-harm behaviors are escalating

High risk: Student reports wanting to die, self-harm methods could be lethal, lacks safety awareness, few protective factors

Means Restriction in School Environment

Means restriction – limiting access to tools that could be used for self-harm – is a crucial safety strategy that needs to be implemented sensitively to avoid feeling punitive.

Classroom considerations:

- Work with teachers to secure or monitor sharp objects (scissors, compasses, craft knives)

- Be mindful of lab equipment in science classes

- Consider modifications to art class activities that involve cutting tools
- Monitor access to cleaning supplies or chemicals

PE and athletics modifications:

- Be aware of potential self-harm in locker rooms or bathrooms
- Monitor for injuries that might be self-inflicted but reported as accidental
- Ensure appropriate supervision during activities where injuries are common

General school environment:

- Check areas where students might find improvised self-harm tools
- Be aware of broken fixtures, sharp edges, or other environmental hazards
- Monitor school supplies that could be misused

Supervision Requirements Determination

The level of supervision needed depends on the severity of self-harm behavior, the student's level of safety awareness, and their willingness to engage in safety planning.

Minimal supervision: Student with good insight, willing to use safety plan, self-harm is infrequent and not severe

- Regular check-ins (2-3 times per day)
- Clear protocols for seeking help
- Monitoring by multiple staff members

Moderate supervision: Student with some safety concerns, escalating behavior, or poor insight

- Frequent check-ins (hourly during high-risk periods)

- Limited time alone, especially in bathrooms or isolated areas

- Direct supervision during potentially triggering activities

Intensive supervision: Student with high safety risk, severe self-harm, or poor safety planning

- Constant adult supervision

- One-on-one aide if necessary

- Possible alternative educational setting until stabilized

- Emergency protocols readily available

Documentation and Reporting

Self-harm incidents require careful documentation that balances thorough record-keeping with student privacy and dignity. Your documentation might be reviewed by administrators, parents, mental health professionals, or even legal authorities, so accuracy and professionalism are crucial.

Mandatory Reporting Considerations

Self-harm behaviors don't automatically trigger mandatory reporting requirements, but certain circumstances do require reporting to child protective services:

Report to CPS when:

- Self-harm appears to be the result of abuse or neglect by caregivers

- Parents refuse to seek necessary medical or mental health treatment for self-harm

- Self-harm is occurring in the context of other abuse or neglect

- Students report that caregivers are encouraging or facilitating self-harm

Don't automatically report:

- Self-harm behaviors alone, without other indicators of abuse or neglect

- Situations where parents are cooperative in seeking treatment

- Cases where appropriate safety planning is in place and effective

When in doubt, consult:

- School administrators

- District legal counsel

- Child protective services for guidance (without identifying the student)

- Mental health professionals involved in the case

FERPA-Compliant Documentation

Your documentation needs to be thorough enough to ensure continuity of care and legal protection, but it must also comply with privacy laws and respect student dignity.

Document objectively:

- Physical description of injuries (location, size, appearance, apparent age)

- Student's exact words about how injuries occurred

- Your observations of emotional state and behavior

- Safety planning steps taken

- Who was notified and when

- Follow-up plans and referrals made

Avoid subjective interpretations:

- Don't speculate about motivation unless the student explicitly states it

- Avoid diagnostic language or psychological interpretations

- Don't document opinions about family dynamics unless directly relevant to safety

- Keep descriptions clinical and professional

Sample documentation format:

Date/Time: 10/15/24, 2:30 PM *Student:* Jane Doe, Grade 10 *Presenting issue:* Multiple linear cuts observed on left forearm during routine health check *Physical assessment:* Approximately 8 superficial cuts, 1-2 inches long, various stages of healing *Student report:* "I cut myself when I feel really stressed out. It helps me feel better." *Safety assessment:* Denies suicidal intent, reports cutting 2-3 times per week for past month *Actions taken:* Wounds cleaned and bandaged, parents contacted, safety plan developed *Referrals:* School counselor appointment scheduled for 10/16/24 *Follow-up:* Daily check-ins scheduled, parent meeting on 10/17/24

Communication with Treatment Providers

If the student is receiving mental health treatment, coordination with their providers is essential for consistent care. However, information sharing must comply with privacy laws and involve appropriate consent.

Information you can share with written parental consent:

- Specific self-harm incidents and their circumstances

- Safety planning strategies that work at school

- Academic or social concerns that might be relevant to treatment

- Medication side effects or issues you observe

- Progress or setbacks you notice in the school setting

Information to request from treatment providers:

- General treatment goals and how you can support them

- Warning signs to watch for that might indicate increased risk

- Specific strategies that work for the student during difficult periods

- Academic accommodations that might be helpful

- Communication protocols for sharing concerns or observations

Re-entry After Self-Harm Incident

When a student returns to school after a self-harm incident – whether they've been out for medical treatment, mental health evaluation, or just needed a day or two off – your re-entry process can set the tone for their ongoing recovery and school success.

Safety Contract Alternatives

Traditional safety contracts ("I promise not to hurt myself") have fallen out of favor because they don't actually prevent self-harm and can damage therapeutic relationships if students can't keep unrealistic promises. Instead, focus on concrete safety planning.

Safety planning elements:

- Specific warning signs that precede urges to self-harm

- Coping strategies to try before resorting to self-harm

- People to contact when feeling urges (specific names and contact methods)

- Ways to make the environment safer (removing or securing potential tools)

- Reasons for living and reasons to stay safe

- Professional contacts for emergency situations

Making safety plans concrete:

- "When I notice that I'm feeling overwhelmed and want to be alone, I will..."
- "Before I hurt myself, I will try these three things..."
- "If those don't work, I will talk to..."
- "I will keep myself safe by..."

Coping Kit Development

Help students develop a personalized collection of tools and strategies they can use instead of self-harm. This kit should be readily accessible and contain items that address the specific functions that self-harm serves for that student.

For students who self-harm for emotional release:

- Stress balls, exercise bands, or other objects to squeeze
- Ice cubes to hold or rub on skin
- Intense physical exercise routines
- Loud music and safe space to scream or cry

For students who self-harm to feel something:

- Strong mints, sour candy, or other intense tastes
- Ice or cold water on skin
- Elastic bands to snap on wrists (gently)
- Intense but safe sensory experiences

For students who self-harm to see blood or injury:

- Red marker to draw on skin
- Ketchup or red paint to simulate blood

- Drawing or writing about feelings instead

For students who self-harm for control:

- Journaling or creative expression
- Making lists or organizing spaces
- Physical activities they can control (push-ups, stretching)
- Breathing exercises or meditation

Peer Response Management

Other students might notice signs of self-harm, and their reactions can either support recovery or create additional problems. You need strategies for managing peer awareness while protecting the student's privacy.

If other students notice and express concern:

- Validate their caring but maintain confidentiality about specifics
- Provide general information about how to support friends who are struggling
- Encourage them to talk to adults if they're worried about someone
- Address any myths or misconceptions about self-harm

If other students react negatively:

- Address bullying or harassment immediately and firmly
- Provide education about mental health to reduce stigma
- Monitor social interactions for the student who self-harms
- Consider involving parents if peer harassment continues

If self-harm appears to be "contagious" among students:

- Increase general mental health awareness and education

- Provide additional screening for at-risk students

- Review social media policies and monitor for concerning content

- Bring in additional mental health resources for the school community

Teaching peer support skills:

- How to recognize when a friend is struggling

- Appropriate ways to offer help and support

- When and how to involve adults

- How to take care of their own mental health when supporting others

Chapter 2.4: Eating Disorder Recognition

Fifteen-year-old Maya hasn't eaten lunch in your cafeteria for three weeks. When you ask her about it, she says she "forgot" or "ate a big breakfast" or "isn't hungry today." Her jeans hang loose on her frame, and her PE teacher mentions she seems dizzy during warm-ups. But Maya's grades are excellent, she's involved in multiple activities, and her parents think she's just going through a growth spurt.

Eating disorders are masters of disguise. They hide behind perfectionism, health consciousness, busy schedules, and even other medical conditions. Students with eating disorders become skilled at deflecting concern, minimizing symptoms, and maintaining the appearance of normalcy even as their bodies and minds are suffering significant damage.

Your school-based perspective gives you unique advantages in recognizing eating disorders. You see students during meals, in various activities, across different emotional states, and over extended periods of time. You can spot patterns that parents might miss and changes that seem gradual but are actually significant.

School-Based Warning Signs

Eating disorders manifest differently in school settings than they do in clinical environments. Students might be able to hide behaviors at home, but the structured nature of school days and the social aspects of school meals create situations where eating disorder symptoms become visible.

Lunchroom Behaviors

The cafeteria is your best laboratory for observing eating behaviors, but you need to know what to look for beyond just "not eating enough."

Restrictive eating patterns:

- Consistently bringing lunch but not eating it, or eating only small portions

- Choosing only "safe" foods (usually low-calorie items like salads, fruits, diet foods)

- Cutting food into unusually small pieces or eating extremely slowly

- Appearing to eat but actually moving food around or hiding it

- Making excuses for not eating: "I ate a huge breakfast," "I'm not feeling well," "I'm saving this for later"

- Avoiding social eating situations or making excuses to leave during lunch

Binge eating indicators:

- Eating unusually large amounts of food very quickly

- Eating alone or secretively, avoiding eating in front of others

- Hoarding food or eating food that belongs to others

- Mood changes after eating (guilt, shame, anxiety)

- Going to bathroom immediately after meals (possible purging)

Purging-related behaviors:

- Frequent bathroom visits after meals

- Smell of vomit in bathrooms

- Excessive use of mouthwash, mints, or gum after eating

- Swollen cheeks or jaw area (from frequent vomiting)

- Dental problems or complaints of sore throat

Other concerning lunchroom behaviors:

- Obsessive calorie counting or reading nutrition labels extensively

- Refusing to eat unless they know exact ingredients or preparation methods

- Extreme anxiety when favorite foods aren't available

- Competitive eating behaviors or encouraging others not to eat

- Teaching other students about calories, "bad" foods, or weight loss

PE Class Avoidance Patterns

Physical education classes reveal eating disorder symptoms that might not be obvious in other settings, particularly around body image, energy levels, and the relationship between food and exercise.

Avoidance strategies:

- Frequent requests to be excused from PE for minor health complaints

- Patterns of illness on PE days or when swimming/changing clothes is required

- Asking to sit out activities that require physical exertion

- Coming to your office during PE with vague complaints

- "Forgetting" PE clothes frequently

Performance-related indicators:

- Dramatic decline in athletic performance or endurance

- Dizziness, fainting, or excessive fatigue during physical activity

- Inability to regulate body temperature (always cold, especially hands and feet)

- Taking much longer to recover from physical activity than peers

- Injuries that heal slowly or occur more frequently than expected

Body image concerns in PE:

- Extreme self-consciousness about changing clothes

- Wearing multiple layers during exercise

- Avoiding activities where body shape might be visible

- Excessive concern about appearance during physical activity

- Comments about feeling "fat" or "disgusting" in athletic clothing

Exercise addiction signs:

- Exercising beyond what's required or appropriate

- Becoming anxious or agitated when unable to exercise

- Exercising despite injury or illness

- Using PE class to "make up for" eating

- Talking about exercise primarily in terms of burning calories or punishment

Bathroom Monitoring Concerns

Bathroom behaviors can provide important clues about purging behaviors, though you need to balance monitoring with respect for privacy.

Signs of purging to watch for:

- Frequent bathroom visits immediately after meals

- Long periods spent in bathroom stalls
- Running water or flushing toilets repeatedly
- Unusual sounds from bathroom stalls
- Students who seem to "disappear" after lunch consistently

Physical evidence you might observe:
- Vomit smell in bathrooms, especially after lunch periods
- Unusual amounts of toilet paper use
- Students emerging from bathrooms with watery eyes or flushed faces
- Frequent complaints of "stomach bugs" or nausea after meals

Behavioral patterns:
- Always using the same bathroom stall
- Becoming defensive or anxious when bathroom access is limited
- Carrying large water bottles or drinks into bathrooms
- Avoiding bathrooms when other students are present

Medical Assessment Priorities

Eating disorders can cause serious medical complications, some of which can be life-threatening. Your medical assessment skills are crucial for determining when eating disorder symptoms require immediate medical attention versus ongoing monitoring and support.

Vital Sign Parameters Requiring Action

Eating disorders affect multiple body systems, and vital sign abnormalities can indicate dangerous medical instability.

Heart rate concerns:

- *Bradycardia (slow heart rate):* Less than 50 beats per minute at rest requires immediate evaluation

- *Tachycardia (fast heart rate):* Over 100 beats per minute at rest, especially if accompanied by other symptoms

- *Irregular heartbeat:* Any rhythm abnormalities or heart palpitations

- *Orthostatic changes:* Heart rate increase of more than 20 beats per minute when standing up

Blood pressure issues:

- *Hypotension:* Systolic BP less than 90 or diastolic less than 60

- *Orthostatic hypotension:* Drop in systolic BP of 20+ points or diastolic of 10+ points when standing

- *Hypertension:* Can occur with certain eating disorder behaviors or medical complications

Temperature regulation:

- *Hypothermia:* Body temperature below 96°F (35.6°C)

- *Inability to maintain normal body temperature*

- *Always feeling cold, especially extremities*

Respiratory concerns:

- *Breathing rate abnormalities:* Too fast, too slow, or irregular patterns

- *Shortness of breath with minimal exertion*

- *Chest pain or difficulty taking deep breaths*

When to Require Medical Clearance for School

Some eating disorder symptoms pose immediate risks that make it unsafe for students to remain in the regular school environment without medical evaluation and clearance.

Immediate medical clearance required:

- Any vital sign abnormalities listed above
- Fainting or near-fainting episodes
- Chest pain or heart palpitations
- Severe dehydration (dry mouth, no urination, extreme thirst)
- Electrolyte imbalance symptoms (muscle weakness, confusion, seizures)
- Significant weight loss (more than 10% of body weight in short period)

Medical clearance recommended within 24-48 hours:

- Persistent dizziness or lightheadedness
- Extreme fatigue that interferes with functioning
- Dental problems that suggest frequent vomiting
- Hair loss, brittle nails, or other signs of malnutrition
- Mood changes that might indicate medical causes
- Sleep disturbances related to eating behaviors

Ongoing medical monitoring needed:

- Regular weight checks if weight loss is occurring
- Periodic vital sign monitoring for students with known eating disorders
- Coordination with healthcare providers about medical stability

- Documentation of any physical symptoms or changes

Activity Restriction Guidelines

Students with eating disorders might need modifications to their physical activity to prevent medical complications while still allowing them to participate in school as normally as possible.

Consider restricting physical activity when:

- Vital signs are abnormal or unstable
- Student reports dizziness, chest pain, or extreme fatigue
- Recent fainting episodes or near-fainting
- Significant dehydration or other medical complications
- Healthcare provider recommends activity restrictions

Modifications rather than complete restrictions:

- Allow rest breaks during PE activities
- Provide alternatives to high-intensity exercises
- Monitor closely during physical activities
- Ensure adequate hydration is available
- Allow students to stop activities if they feel unwell

Family Communication Strategies

Talking to families about eating disorder concerns is one of the most delicate conversations you'll have as a school nurse. Parents might be defensive, in denial, or overwhelmed. They might blame themselves, minimize the problem, or react with anger. Your approach can determine whether the family becomes a partner in recovery or creates additional barriers to getting help.

Approaching Resistant Parents

Some parents have difficulty accepting that their child might have an eating disorder. This resistance often comes from fear, stigma, or lack of understanding about eating disorders.

Common parental reactions and responses:

- *"She's just being healthy/watching her weight"* – Provide education about the difference between healthy eating and eating disorder behaviors

- *"He's always been a picky eater"* – Help them see changes over time and the impact on functioning

- *"We don't have eating disorders in our family"* – Explain that eating disorders can affect anyone regardless of family history

- *"She's not thin enough to have an eating disorder"* – Educate about different types of eating disorders and that weight isn't the only indicator

Strategies for resistant families:

- Lead with concern and care, not accusations

- Use specific observations rather than diagnostic labels initially

- Focus on changes you've noticed rather than absolute behaviors

- Emphasize that early intervention leads to better outcomes

- Offer to provide educational resources about eating disorders

- Suggest starting with their family doctor rather than immediately seeking specialized treatment

Cultural Considerations in Eating Behaviors

Cultural background significantly influences attitudes about food, body image, and eating behaviors. What seems concerning in one cultural context might be normal in another, and vice versa.

Cultural factors to consider:

- Traditional foods and eating patterns that might seem restrictive to outsiders

- Cultural attitudes about body size and shape (some cultures value larger body sizes)

- Religious or cultural fasting practices that might affect eating patterns

- Family dynamics around food preparation, meal times, and eating together

- Economic factors that might influence food availability or choices

- Immigration experiences that might have affected relationships with food

Culturally responsive approaches:

- Ask about family traditions and cultural practices around food

- Involve cultural liaisons or community leaders when appropriate

- Respect cultural values while still addressing health concerns

- Understand that eating disorder treatment might need cultural adaptations

- Be aware of language barriers that might affect communication about eating and body image

Resource Provision Protocols

Families need concrete information and resources, but they also need guidance about how to navigate the complex world of eating disorder treatment.

Initial resources to provide:

- Educational materials about eating disorders (in appropriate languages)
- Local treatment providers who specialize in eating disorders
- Support groups for families dealing with eating disorders
- Books, websites, or other reliable information sources
- Information about insurance coverage for eating disorder treatment

Help families understand:

- Different levels of eating disorder treatment (outpatient, intensive outpatient, residential)
- What to look for in treatment providers
- How to support recovery at home without becoming the "food police"
- Warning signs that indicate the need for higher level of care
- How to handle resistance from their child about seeking treatment

Chapter 2.5: Psychosis and Severe Mental Illness

The first signs are often subtle. A previously social student begins sitting alone, talking to themselves under their breath. A high achiever starts writing incomprehensible essays filled with strange connections between unrelated ideas. A friendly teenager becomes suspicious and fearful, convinced that classmates are plotting against them.

Early psychosis in adolescents can be terrifying for everyone involved – the student, their family, their teachers, and you. Unlike depression or anxiety, which most people can relate to on some level, psychosis feels foreign and frightening. Students experiencing psychotic symptoms often don't recognize that their perceptions and thoughts aren't based in reality, making them resistant to help and difficult to support.

Your role in recognizing early psychosis could literally change the trajectory of a young person's life. Early intervention in psychotic disorders dramatically improves long-term outcomes, but the average time between symptom onset and appropriate treatment is still several years. You might be the first person to recognize that a student's changing behavior represents something more serious than typical teenage moodiness or academic stress.

Early Psychosis Recognition

Psychosis doesn't usually appear suddenly. Most young people experience a prodromal period – weeks or months of gradual changes that precede the onset of frank psychotic symptoms. During this prodromal phase, intervention can sometimes prevent progression to full psychosis or significantly reduce its severity.

Prodromal Symptoms in Adolescents

The early warning signs of psychosis in teenagers often look like other mental health problems or normal adolescent behavior, which is why they're frequently missed or misinterpreted.

Cognitive changes:

- Difficulty concentrating that's more severe than typical ADHD or anxiety

- Problems with memory, especially working memory (holding information in mind)

- Disorganized thinking that shows up in speech or writing

- Declining academic performance despite previous good functioning

- Trouble following conversations or losing track of what others are saying

- Difficulty making decisions, even about simple things

Perceptual changes:

- Reports of hearing voices or sounds that others don't hear (but still recognizing these might not be real)

- Seeing shadows, lights, or movements in peripheral vision

- Feeling like things look different somehow – brighter, dimmer, or distorted

- Increased sensitivity to sounds, lights, or textures

- Feeling disconnected from their body or like they're watching themselves from outside

Social and emotional changes:

- Withdrawal from friends and family members

- Losing interest in activities they previously enjoyed

- Flat or inappropriate emotional responses

- Increased anxiety, especially social anxiety or paranoid fears

- Mood swings that seem more extreme than typical teenage emotions

- Feeling like other people are different somehow or can't be trusted

Behavioral changes:

- Sleep pattern disruptions (staying up all night, sleeping during the day)

- Personal hygiene deterioration

- Strange or ritualistic behaviors

- Talking to themselves more than usual

- Writing or drawing content that seems bizarre or concerning

- Expressing unusual beliefs or interests that seem disconnected from reality

Differentiating from Substance Use

Substance use, particularly marijuana, stimulants, and hallucinogens, can cause symptoms that look very similar to early psychosis. Some students develop substance-induced psychotic episodes that resolve when they stop using, while others use substances to self-medicate psychotic symptoms that were already developing.

Clues that suggest primary psychosis rather than substance-induced symptoms:

- Symptoms persist during periods when student reports not using substances

- Symptoms began before any substance use or with very minimal use

- Family history of psychotic disorders or other serious mental illness

- Gradual onset of symptoms over weeks or months rather than acute episodes

- Symptoms are present throughout the day, not just when using or withdrawing from substances

Clues that suggest substance-induced psychosis:

- Symptoms only occur in conjunction with substance use

- Rapid onset of symptoms after beginning substance use

- Symptoms resolve completely when substances are discontinued

- Student has insight that symptoms might be related to substance use

- No family history of psychotic disorders

Important considerations:

- Substance use and psychosis can coexist – students with developing psychotic disorders often self-medicate with drugs or alcohol

- Some students develop persistent psychotic symptoms after substance use that don't resolve even with sobriety

- Certain substances (particularly synthetic drugs and high-potency marijuana) can trigger psychotic episodes in vulnerable individuals

Academic and Social Function Changes

The impact of developing psychosis on school functioning is often one of the most noticeable early signs, especially for students who were previously successful academically and socially.

Academic function decline:

- Grades dropping across multiple subjects, not just one difficult class

- Assignments becoming disorganized, tangential, or incomprehensible

- Inability to follow multi-step directions or complete complex tasks

- Difficulty participating in class discussions or group work

- Teachers reporting the student seems "not present" or "in their own world"

- Previously verbal students becoming silent or giving very brief responses

Social function changes:

- Withdrawal from friend groups and social activities

- Peers reporting the student is "acting weird" or "different"

- Difficulty maintaining conversations or seeming to respond to things others can't hear or see

- Increased conflicts with peers or authority figures

- Paranoid concerns about other students or teachers

- Loss of social skills that were previously well-developed

Immediate Safety Protocols

When you suspect a student might be experiencing psychotic symptoms, your immediate priorities are ensuring their safety and the safety of others, while also preserving your therapeutic relationship and avoiding actions that increase their fear or paranoia.

Environmental Modification

Students experiencing psychosis often feel overwhelmed by sensory input and may be more likely to misinterpret neutral environmental cues as threatening.

Create a calming environment:

- Move to a quiet, private space with minimal distractions
- Reduce lighting if possible (bright lights can feel overwhelming)
- Minimize background noise and interruptions
- Keep the space uncluttered and simple
- Ensure there are no objects that could be used as weapons if the student becomes agitated

Positioning and approach:

- Stay at eye level rather than standing over the student
- Maintain some distance – don't crowd or corner them
- Keep your hands visible and avoid sudden movements
- Position yourself between the student and the door (for your safety) but don't block their exit
- Remove any potential triggers from the environment

Communication Strategies for Confused Students

How you talk to a student experiencing psychotic symptoms can either help them feel safer and more grounded or increase their confusion and paranoia.

Effective communication strategies:

- Speak slowly, clearly, and simply – use short sentences

- Use the student's name frequently to help them stay oriented

- Avoid arguing with or directly contradicting their perceptions

- Don't pretend to see or hear things you don't, but don't call them "crazy" either

- Focus on their feelings rather than the reality of their perceptions: "That sounds really frightening" rather than "That's not real"

- Repeat important information multiple times

- Check for understanding frequently: "Do you understand what I'm saying?"

Phrases that help:

- "You're safe here with me"

- "I'm here to help you"

- "I can see this is really distressing for you"

- "Let's figure this out together"

- "What would help you feel safer right now?"

Avoid these approaches:

- "You're just imagining things"

- "That's not real" or "You're being paranoid"

- Laughing at or dismissing their concerns

- Making promises you can't keep

- Overwhelming them with questions or complex explanations

- Using medical or psychiatric terminology

When to Call Emergency Services

Determining when psychotic symptoms require emergency intervention can be challenging, but certain situations always warrant immediate professional help.

Call 911 or emergency services immediately for:

- Any threats of violence toward self or others
- Severely disorganized behavior that poses immediate safety risks
- Inability to care for basic safety needs (wandering into traffic, not recognizing dangers)
- Catatonic symptoms (not moving, not responding to stimuli)
- Medical emergency symptoms in conjunction with psychosis
- Command hallucinations telling the student to hurt themselves or others

Consider emergency evaluation for:

- First episode of clear psychotic symptoms
- Rapid deterioration in functioning over days or weeks
- Inability to distinguish reality from hallucinations or delusions
- Extreme agitation or terror related to psychotic symptoms
- Refusal to eat or drink due to paranoid fears
- Parents unable to manage the student safely at home

Can usually manage with urgent (same-day) referral:

- Mild psychotic symptoms with good insight
- Gradual onset of symptoms over weeks or months
- Student is cooperative and not expressing safety concerns

- Family is available and able to provide support

- Student has some ability to reality-test their experiences

Coordination with Mental Health Services

Students experiencing psychosis need specialized mental health care that goes beyond what schools can provide. Your role becomes coordinating care, facilitating communication between providers and school staff, and ensuring continuity of support.

Hospital Liaison Protocols

When students are hospitalized for psychiatric evaluation or treatment, maintaining communication helps ensure smooth transitions back to school.

Information to provide to hospital staff:

- Specific symptoms and behaviors you observed at school

- Timeline of symptom development and changes

- Academic and social functioning before and during symptom onset

- Any triggers or patterns you've noticed

- Student's strengths and effective coping strategies

- Family dynamics and support system information

Information to request from hospital:

- Diagnosis and treatment recommendations

- Medications and potential side effects to monitor

- Activity restrictions or accommodations needed

- Warning signs of symptom worsening

- Timeline for follow-up and ongoing treatment

Medication Management in Schools

Students with psychotic disorders often require antipsychotic medications that can have significant side effects affecting their ability to function in school.

Common side effects to monitor:

- Sedation or drowsiness (especially in morning classes)
- Movement side effects (tremor, stiffness, restlessness)
- Weight gain and metabolic changes
- Dizziness or orthostatic hypotension
- Cognitive dulling or difficulty concentrating
- Temperature regulation problems

Accommodation considerations:

- Schedule adjustments if medications cause morning sedation
- Frequent breaks for students experiencing restlessness
- Modified PE requirements if weight gain or movement issues occur
- Additional time for assignments if cognitive processing is slowed
- Temperature control accommodations if needed
- Snack breaks if medications affect blood sugar

Communication with prescribing providers:

- Report side effects or concerns promptly
- Document any changes in school functioning
- Provide feedback about medication effectiveness

- Coordinate timing of medication administration if given at school

Re-integration Planning

Students returning to school after psychotic episodes need carefully planned re-integration that balances academic expectations with mental health needs.

Academic considerations:

- Modified course load if cognitive symptoms are present
- Extended time for assignments and tests
- Quiet testing environment to reduce distractions
- Permission to leave class if symptoms worsen
- Alternative assessment methods if traditional tests are overwhelming
- Gradual increase in academic expectations as functioning improves

Social considerations:

- Peer education (with family consent) to reduce stigma and misunderstanding
- Structured social interactions rather than unstructured free time initially
- Support for rebuilding friendships that might have been affected
- Monitoring for bullying or social isolation
- Connection with understanding peers or mentors
- Gradual reintroduction to extracurricular activities

Safety planning:

- Identify early warning signs of symptom recurrence

- Create protocols for what to do if symptoms return at school

- Establish communication systems between home, school, and treatment providers

- Plan for medication compliance and monitoring

- Develop crisis intervention procedures specific to the student's needs

Long-term support planning:

- Regular mental health check-ins (weekly initially, then less frequent)

- Coordination with ongoing outpatient treatment

- Academic planning that accounts for the episodic nature of psychotic disorders

- Vocational planning and transition services for older students

- Family education and support services

- Connection with community resources and support groups

Practical Tools for Implementation

The complexity of recognizing and responding to various mental health presentations requires practical tools that help you make quick, accurate decisions while ensuring comprehensive care.

Tear-out Flowchart Cards for Each Condition

Create wallet-sized cards for each major mental health condition that include:

Anxiety Card:

- Quick recognition signs (physical symptoms, avoidance patterns)

- Immediate intervention steps (grounding techniques, safe space protocols)
- Escalation indicators (when to call parents, when to call 911)
- Follow-up requirements

Depression Card:

- Age-specific warning signs
- Safety assessment questions
- PHQ-9 score interpretation and actions
- Referral and monitoring protocols

Self-Harm Card:

- Types of self-harm behaviors
- Medical assessment priorities
- Safety planning steps
- Documentation requirements

Eating Disorder Card:

- School-based warning signs
- Vital sign parameters requiring action
- Family communication strategies
- Medical clearance guidelines

Psychosis Card:

- Prodromal symptoms by category
- Communication strategies for confused students
- Emergency intervention criteria
- Coordination protocols

Mobile App with Interactive Decision Trees

A smartphone app could provide instant access to decision-making support:

Features to include:

- Symptom checkers that guide you through assessment questions

- Automatic score calculation for screening tools

- Quick access to emergency contacts and protocols

- Documentation templates that can be completed on the phone

- Reminder systems for follow-up appointments and check-ins

- Resource databases with local provider information

Decision tree examples:

- Student reports sadness → Assess duration and severity → Check safety → Determine appropriate intervention level → Document and follow up

- Student exhibits anxiety symptoms → Identify type of anxiety → Apply appropriate de-escalation technique → Assess need for parent contact → Plan return to class or further intervention

Warning Sign Posters for Office

Visual reminders help you and other staff quickly recognize concerning symptoms:

Elementary warning signs poster:

- Behavioral regression indicators

- Physical symptom red flags

- Social withdrawal signs

- Academic performance changes

Middle school warning signs poster:

- Peer relationship disruption patterns
- Identity development concerns
- Academic motivation changes
- Risk-taking behavior indicators

High school warning signs poster:

- Substance use warning signs
- Severe depression indicators
- Eating disorder symptoms
- Psychosis early warning signs

Quick-Reference Intervention Cards

Laminated cards with step-by-step protocols for common situations:

Panic attack intervention card:

- 10-step protocol with timing guidelines
- Breathing technique instructions
- When to call for medical help
- Documentation requirements

Suicide risk assessment card:

- ASQ questions and follow-up protocols
- Safety planning steps
- Parent notification requirements
- Emergency contact procedures

Self-harm response card:

- Medical assessment priorities

- Safety planning components

- Documentation templates

- Follow-up scheduling guidelines

Building Your Mental Health Response System

You now have detailed knowledge about recognizing and responding to the most common and serious mental health presentations you'll encounter in schools. But knowledge without a systematic approach can feel overwhelming when you're facing multiple students with different needs on the same day.

Your red flag flowcharts aren't just tools – they're your early warning system that helps you identify problems before they become crises, respond appropriately to different levels of severity, and ensure that no student falls through the cracks. The key is consistent use and regular practice with these protocols until they become second nature.

Most importantly, you're not expected to be a mental health therapist. Your role is to recognize, respond appropriately, connect students with appropriate resources, and provide ongoing support within the school setting. These flowcharts help you stay within your scope of practice while still providing the comprehensive care that students need and deserve.

The investment you make in mastering these assessment and intervention protocols will pay dividends not just in individual student outcomes, but in creating a school culture where mental health is taken seriously, addressed promptly, and supported comprehensively. You're building more than just clinical skills – you're building a safety net that could literally save lives.

Section 3: Crisis Response Protocols

Chapter 3.1: Suicidal Ideation Management

It's 10:47 AM on a Tuesday when 16-year-old Alex sits across from you in your office, staring at the floor. "I answered yes to one of those questions on the health screening," they say quietly. "The one about wishing I was dead." Your heart rate increases slightly, but your voice stays calm and steady. "Thank you for telling me that, Alex. I'm really glad you trusted me with this information."

This moment – when a student discloses suicidal thoughts – represents one of the most critical situations you'll face as a school nurse. Your response in the next few minutes could literally save a life. But it's also when your training, protocols, and preparation matter most. You don't have time to figure out what to do. You need to know exactly what steps to take, in what order, and why each step matters.

Suicidal ideation isn't rare among students. Research indicates that nearly 20% of high school students seriously consider suicide each year, and about 9% make an attempt. But here's what gives you hope: most suicidal crises are temporary. Students who receive appropriate intervention during suicidal episodes often go on to live full, productive lives. Your skilled response can be the bridge that carries them from their darkest moment to a place of safety and healing.

Immediate Response Protocol

When a student discloses suicidal thoughts or screens positive for suicide risk, every second matters. But rushing or panicking helps no one. Your immediate response needs to be swift, systematic, and calm.

The First 60 Seconds: Safety and Rapport

Your initial response sets the tone for everything that follows. Students who disclose suicidal thoughts are taking an enormous risk – they're revealing their most painful and frightening thoughts to an adult who might react with alarm, judgment, or immediate action that takes control away from them.

Immediate verbal responses that build rapport:

- "Thank you for trusting me with this information"
- "I'm really glad you told me how you're feeling"
- "You did the right thing by letting me know"
- "I can see this took courage to share"

What NOT to say in the first 60 seconds:

- "Everything will be okay" (you don't know that yet)
- "You have so much to live for" (minimizes their pain)
- "How could you think that?" (creates shame)
- "Suicide is never the answer" (sounds dismissive)
- "I have to call your parents right now" (increases panic)

Physical positioning and environment:

- Move to a private space immediately if you're not already there
- Sit at eye level rather than standing over the student
- Remove any obvious means of harm from immediate reach
- Ensure the door is closed but not locked
- Position yourself between the student and the door (for safety) without making them feel trapped

Assess immediate safety in the first 60 seconds:

- Are they agitated, actively distressed, or calm?
- Do they seem coherent and able to engage in conversation?

- Are they expressing immediate intent to harm themselves right now?

- Do they have any visible injuries or signs of recent self-harm?

ASQ Positive Screen Response Algorithm

The Ask Suicide-Screening Questions (ASQ) provides a standardized approach for responding to positive suicide screens. This algorithm ensures you don't miss critical steps while managing your own anxiety about the situation.

Step 1: Acknowledge and validate (already covered in first 60 seconds)

Step 2: Ask follow-up questions immediately:

- "Can you tell me more about these thoughts?"

- "When did you start having thoughts about dying?"

- "Have you thought about how you might hurt yourself?"

- "Do you have access to [whatever method they mention]?"

- "What has kept you safe so far?"

Step 3: Assess immediacy of risk:

- *Immediate risk:* Student has plan, means, and intent to harm themselves today

- *High risk:* Student has thoughts with some planning but no immediate intent

- *Moderate risk:* Student has thoughts but good reality testing and safety awareness

Step 4: Implement appropriate safety measures:

- *Immediate risk:* Do not leave alone, consider calling 911, immediate parent contact

- *High risk:* Constant supervision, immediate professional evaluation, same-day safety planning

- *Moderate risk:* Enhanced monitoring, safety planning, professional referral within 24-48 hours

Step 5: Document everything:

- Exact words the student used

- Your assessment of risk level

- Safety measures implemented

- Who you contacted and when

- Student's response to interventions

Supervision and Means Restriction

Once you identify suicide risk, you must ensure the student's immediate physical safety while maintaining therapeutic rapport.

Supervision protocols by risk level:

Immediate/High Risk:

- Student must be within arm's reach of a responsible adult at all times

- Bathroom breaks require adult escort or door left open

- No access to potential means of harm (sharp objects, medications, cleaning supplies)

- Multiple staff members should be aware of the situation

- Consider one-on-one aide if needed

Moderate Risk:

- Adult supervision with line of sight at all times

- Check-ins every 15-30 minutes minimum

- Restricted access to potential means of harm

- Clear protocols for movement between locations

- Other staff alerted to watch for concerning changes

Lower Risk:

- Adult knowledge of whereabouts at all times

- Check-ins every hour

- General means restriction (remove obvious risks)

- Clear communication about where student can and cannot go

Means restriction in school environment:

- Secure or remove sharp objects (scissors, craft knives, broken glass)

- Monitor access to cleaning supplies or chemicals

- Be aware of potential environmental hazards (high places, heavy objects)

- Consider removal from potentially triggering classes (chemistry lab, shop class)

- Restrict access to medications in nurse's office

Never Leave Alone Protocols

The "never leave alone" protocol is non-negotiable for students at immediate or high risk for suicide, but it requires careful implementation to avoid feeling punitive.

How to implement continuous supervision:

- Explain to the student why you're staying close: "I need to make sure you're safe right now"

- If you must leave, arrange for another trusted adult to take your place

- During transitions, maintain visual contact and close proximity

- Use bathroom buddy system or leave door ajar during bathroom use

- Ensure sleeping supervision if student needs to rest

Who can provide supervision:

- School nurses, counselors, social workers, or administrators

- Trained teachers or staff members (with brief orientation about what to watch for)

- Mental health professionals if available

- Trusted adult volunteers in emergency situations (with staff oversight)

What supervisors should watch for:

- Signs of increasing agitation or distress

- Attempts to access potential means of harm

- Statements about wanting to hurt themselves

- Attempts to isolate or escape supervision

- Changes in mood, energy, or coherence

Risk Stratification

Not all suicidal thoughts carry the same level of immediate danger. Your ability to quickly and accurately assess risk level determines how urgently you need to respond and what interventions are most appropriate.

Low, Moderate, and High Risk Indicators

Low Risk Indicators:

106

- Student reports occasional thoughts of death but no specific plans

- Good reality testing and safety awareness ("I would never actually do it")

- Strong protective factors (family connections, future goals, religious beliefs)

- Willing to engage in safety planning

- No access to lethal means

- No history of suicide attempts

- Adequate support system

- Able to identify reasons for living

Typical low-risk statement: "Sometimes I think about what it would be like if I wasn't here, but I know I wouldn't actually hurt myself because of my family."

Moderate Risk Indicators:

- Specific thoughts about death or self-harm but no definite plans

- Some planning behavior but low likelihood of immediate action

- Mixed protective and risk factors

- Ambivalent about living ("I don't really want to die, but I can't keep feeling this way")

- Limited access to lethal means

- Some social support but may feel disconnected

- Previous episodes of suicidal thinking without action

Typical moderate-risk statement: "I think about taking pills or something, but I don't really want to die. I just want the pain to stop."

High Risk Indicators:

- Specific plan for self-harm with access to means
- Recent suicide attempt or aborted attempt
- Giving away possessions or saying goodbye
- Sudden improvement in mood after period of depression (may indicate decision has been made)
- Substance use combined with suicidal thoughts
- History of impulsive behavior
- Social isolation or recent losses
- Expression of hopelessness about the future

Typical high-risk statement: "I'm going to take my dad's gun tonight after everyone goes to sleep. I've got it all figured out."

C-SSRS Triage Version Implementation

The Columbia Suicide Severity Rating Scale triage version provides a structured way to assess suicide risk that goes beyond simple yes/no questions.

Suicidal Ideation Assessment (ask in order, stop when you get to "yes"):

Level 1 - Wish to be Dead: "Have you wished you were dead or wished you could go to sleep and not wake up?"

Level 2 - Suicidal Thoughts: "Have you actually had thoughts of killing yourself?"

Level 3 - Suicidal Thoughts with Method: "Have you thought about how you might kill yourself?"

Level 4 - Suicidal Intent: "Have you had these thoughts and had some intention of acting on them?"

Level 5 - Suicidal Intent with Plan: "Have you started to work out or worked out the details of how to kill yourself?"

Suicidal Behavior Assessment:

- "Have you ever made a suicide attempt?"

- "Have you ever done anything, started to do anything, or prepared to do anything to end your life?"

- "Have you ever done anything to hurt yourself without wanting to die?"

Risk level based on C-SSRS results:

- *Levels 1-2 with no behavior:* Usually lower risk, requires monitoring and support

- *Levels 3-4:* Moderate to high risk, requires immediate safety planning and professional evaluation

- *Level 5 or any recent behavior:* High risk, requires immediate intervention and likely emergency evaluation

Documentation Requirements for Each Level

Your documentation must be thorough enough to support clinical decision-making and legal protection while being completed efficiently during crisis situations.

Low Risk Documentation:

- Date, time, setting of assessment

- Specific screening tool results

- Student's exact words about suicidal thoughts

- Protective factors identified

- Safety plan developed

- Parent notification and response

- Follow-up appointments scheduled

- Student's agreement with safety plan

Sample entry: "Student endorsed occasional thoughts of death on PHQ-9 screening but denies specific plans or intent. States 'sometimes I think about not being here but I would never hurt myself because of my little sister.' Strong family connections, involved in theater program. Safety plan developed focusing on talking to mom when feeling overwhelmed. Parents contacted and will follow up with pediatrician. Next check-in scheduled for tomorrow."

Moderate Risk Documentation:

- Everything from low risk, plus:

- Detailed risk assessment including C-SSRS results

- Specific safety measures implemented

- Staff members notified and their roles

- Professional referrals made

- Frequency of follow-up planned

- Any environmental modifications made

High Risk Documentation:

- Everything from moderate risk, plus:

- Minute-by-minute timeline of crisis intervention

- Exact quotes about plans, means, and intent

- Emergency contacts made (times, who spoke, outcomes)

- Law enforcement involvement if applicable

- Hospital referrals or emergency evaluations

- Continuous supervision protocols implemented

- Detailed safety planning with specific steps

Parent Notification Procedures

Contacting parents about their child's suicidal thoughts is one of the most difficult conversations you'll have, but it's also one of the most important. Your approach can determine whether parents become allies in their child's recovery or create additional barriers to getting help.

Legal Requirements by Risk Level

Understanding your legal obligations helps you navigate the complex balance between student confidentiality and safety requirements.

Immediate notification required (same day):

- Any immediate or high risk suicide assessment

- Student has made recent suicide attempt

- Student has specific plan with access to means

- Student is actively expressing intent to harm themselves

- Professional evaluation recommends immediate parent involvement

Notification recommended within 24 hours:

- Moderate risk assessments

- Significant change in previously identified student's risk level

- Safety planning requires parent involvement to be effective

- Student requests parent involvement

- Professional treatment recommendations require parent consent

Consider student input before notification:

- Low risk assessments in older teens (16-18) with good judgment

- Situations where family conflict may be contributing to suicidal thoughts

- When student demonstrates good safety awareness and has other supports

- Cases where building therapeutic rapport first might improve outcomes

Never notify parents (rare exceptions):

- When parent/family abuse is suspected cause of suicidal thoughts

- When notification would significantly increase risk to student

- When legal consultation advises otherwise

- When custody issues complicate notification (requires legal guidance)

Scripts for Difficult Conversations

How you communicate with parents about suicide risk affects their ability to respond helpfully rather than with panic or denial.

Opening script for high-risk situations: "Hello, Mrs. Smith. This is Sarah Johnson, the school nurse at Lincoln High. I need to talk with you about Alex. They came to see me today and shared some concerning thoughts about wanting to hurt themselves. I want you to know that Alex is safe right now and is here with me in my office, but I'm worried about their safety and think they need immediate professional help."

For moderate-risk situations: "Hi, Mr. Garcia. This is calling from school about Maria. During a routine mental health screening today,

Maria shared that she's been having some thoughts about death and not wanting to be alive. She's not in immediate danger, but I'm concerned about her and think it would be helpful for you to know what's happening so we can work together to get her some support."

For resistant or denying parents: "I understand this is shocking and hard to hear. Many parents feel that way when they first learn about their child's suicidal thoughts. What's important right now is that Alex trusted us enough to share how they're feeling, and that means we have an opportunity to help them before things get worse."

When Parents Refuse Intervention

Sometimes parents minimize, deny, or refuse to seek appropriate help for their suicidal child. This puts you in a difficult position legally and ethically.

Common parental responses and your options:

"They're just being dramatic/attention-seeking":

- Provide education about suicide myths
- Explain that attention-seeking behavior often indicates genuine distress
- Emphasize that suicidal behavior should always be taken seriously
- Document their response and continue monitoring student

"We'll handle this at home":

- Assess whether parents have adequate resources and understanding
- Provide specific guidance about home safety measures
- Require specific follow-up timeline
- Document agreement and follow up as promised

"We don't believe in therapy/medication":

- Respect cultural/religious values while emphasizing safety
- Provide information about various types of help available
- Suggest starting with family doctor or spiritual counselor
- Focus on immediate safety rather than long-term treatment initially

When refusal creates safety concerns:

- Consult with administrators and legal counsel
- Consider mandatory reporting if refusal constitutes neglect
- Increase school-based monitoring and support
- Document all interactions thoroughly
- Consider involving child protective services in extreme cases

Mandated Reporting Triggers

Suicidal ideation itself doesn't automatically trigger mandatory reporting, but certain circumstances do require reporting to child protective services.

Report when:

- Parents refuse to seek necessary emergency mental health evaluation for high-risk child
- Suicidal thoughts appear related to abuse or neglect by caregivers
- Parent's response to child's suicidal crisis involves threats, punishment, or abandonment
- Student reports that parents are encouraging self-harm or expressing wish that child would die
- Family situation appears to be actively increasing suicide risk

Document before reporting:

- Specific evidence of neglect or abuse
- Parents' exact response to notification about suicide risk
- Student's statements about family dynamics
- Professional recommendations that parents are refusing
- Other evidence that child's safety is being compromised by parental response

Consult before reporting:

- School administrators
- District legal counsel
- Mental health professionals involved in case
- Child protective services (for guidance without identifying student)

Crisis Team Activation

No school nurse should handle suicidal students alone. Crisis situations require coordinated team responses that ensure student safety while managing the multiple tasks involved in crisis intervention.

Who to Call and When

Different levels of crisis require different team members and different urgency of response.

Immediate crisis team activation (call right now):

- Student expressing immediate intent to harm themselves
- Student has made suicide attempt at school
- Student with access to means and specific plan

- Student who has become agitated, disoriented, or uncooperative during assessment
- Any situation where you feel the student's safety is in immediate jeopardy

Crisis team members to contact immediately:

- School principal or designated administrator
- School counselor or social worker
- School psychologist if available
- District crisis intervention team if one exists

Urgent activation (within 1 hour):

- High-risk suicide assessment requiring professional evaluation
- Parents cannot be reached or are uncooperative
- Student requires emergency mental health services
- Situation requires coordinated safety planning involving multiple staff

Same-day activation:

- Moderate risk assessments requiring team support
- Complex family situations requiring administrative guidance
- Need for ongoing safety monitoring involving multiple staff
- Coordination of mental health referrals

Information to Gather Before Calling

Being prepared when you contact crisis team members helps them respond more effectively and saves precious time during emergencies.

Essential information to have ready:

- Student's full name, grade, and student ID number
- Current location and who is supervising them
- Brief summary of suicide risk assessment results
- Current safety measures in place
- Parent contact information and whether they've been notified
- Any immediate safety concerns or behaviors observed
- Time crisis began and timeline of your interventions

Additional helpful information:
- Student's mental health history if known
- Previous suicide attempts or concerning episodes
- Current medications or medical conditions
- Family situation and support system
- Academic and social functioning recent changes
- Substance use concerns if relevant

Questions to ask crisis team members:
- What additional safety measures should be implemented?
- Who else needs to be notified and in what order?
- What is the timeline for professional evaluation?
- How should we handle the student's academic schedule?
- What follow-up responsibilities do I have?

Handoff Communication Protocols

When transferring care of a suicidal student to other professionals, clear communication prevents dangerous gaps in supervision and ensures continuity of care.

Transfer to mental health professional: "I'm transferring care of Alex, a 16-year-old junior, who has been with me since 10:45 AM after positive suicide screening. They reported thoughts of taking pills, moderate planning, but no immediate intent. Parents notified and en route. Student has been cooperative, no agitation, denies current intent but requires ongoing safety monitoring. I've implemented 1:1 supervision and means restriction. Here's my documentation and assessment."

Transfer to emergency services: "We need emergency evaluation for Maria, a 15-year-old sophomore, with immediate suicide risk. She has specific plan to hang herself tonight, has access to means, and is expressing firm intent. Parents notified, father will meet at hospital. Student is cooperative but requires continuous supervision. No medical issues, takes no medications. I'm sending documentation and can provide additional information as needed."

Transfer to administrator: "I need administrative support for ongoing crisis management with 17-year-old David. He has moderate suicide risk, parents are refusing professional evaluation, and he'll need enhanced safety monitoring for the remainder of the school day. I've completed risk assessment and safety planning, but need help coordinating supervision and addressing parent refusal."

Safety Planning in Schools

Safety planning is a collaborative process that helps students identify warning signs, coping strategies, and sources of support they can use when suicidal thoughts become intense. School-based safety plans need to be practical, specific, and easily accessible to students during school hours.

Developing Individualized Safety Plans

Effective safety plans are highly specific to each student's triggers, coping strategies, and support system. Generic safety plans don't work because they don't address the unique factors that influence each student's suicidal thoughts.

Step 1: Identify warning signs Work with the student to identify what happens internally and externally before suicidal thoughts become intense.

Internal warning signs might include:

- Specific thoughts ("everyone would be better off without me")
- Emotions (overwhelming sadness, numbness, anger)
- Physical sensations (chest tightness, difficulty breathing)
- Behaviors (isolating, not eating, staying up late)

External warning signs might include:

- Stressful events (failed test, friendship conflict, family problems)
- Times or places that are difficult (Sunday nights, empty hallways)
- Seasonal patterns (dark months, anniversary dates)

Step 2: Personal coping strategies Help students identify activities they can do independently to manage difficult emotions and thoughts.

Effective school-based coping strategies:

- Physical activities (going for walk, doing push-ups, squeezing stress ball)
- Creative outlets (drawing, writing, listening to music)
- Mindfulness techniques (breathing exercises, grounding techniques)
- Distraction activities (puzzles, games, helping others)

- Self-care activities (washing face, getting drink of water, stepping outside)

Step 3: People and social settings that provide distraction or support Identify specific people at school and home who can provide support, and specific social environments that help the student feel better.

School support people:

- Trusted teachers, counselors, coaches, or staff members
- Specific friends who provide positive support
- Adult mentors or tutors
- Extracurricular activity leaders

Social settings that help:

- Specific classes or activities where student feels competent
- Places in school that feel safe and calming
- Friend groups or social activities that provide connection

Step 4: People to ask for help when coping strategies aren't working Create a hierarchy of people to contact when personal coping isn't sufficient.

First line contacts (for less severe distress):

- Trusted friend or peer supporter
- Specific teacher or coach the student feels comfortable with
- School counselor for routine support

Second line contacts (for more intense suicidal thoughts):

- School nurse or mental health professional
- Specific family members who respond helpfully

- Mental health treatment providers if involved

Crisis contacts (for immediate danger):

- Parents or guardians with specific phone numbers
- Emergency mental health services
- Crisis hotlines with specific numbers pre-programmed

Step 5: Making the environment safer Identify specific steps to remove or limit access to means of self-harm.

At school:

- Avoiding certain areas during difficult times
- Asking to have potentially harmful objects secured
- Requesting modified assignments that don't involve triggers
- Planning for safe transitions between classes

At home:

- Specific agreements with family about securing means
- Plans for staying connected with family during difficult periods
- Environmental modifications that support safety

Identifying Safe Staff Members

Not every staff member is appropriate for providing support to suicidal students. You need to identify and prepare specific individuals who can serve as safe contacts and backup support.

Qualities of safe staff members:

- Calm demeanor and ability to manage their own anxiety about suicide

- Good listening skills and ability to avoid lecturing or problem-solving
- Understanding of confidentiality requirements and limits
- Flexibility to provide support when needed
- Reliable presence at school (not frequently absent)
- Existing positive relationship with student when possible

Staff members to approach:

- School counselors, social workers, psychologists
- Administrators who have received mental health training
- Teachers who have expressed interest in student mental health
- Coaches or activity sponsors who know the student well
- Support staff (secretaries, custodians) who students connect with

Training safe staff members:

- Brief overview of student's situation (with appropriate consent)
- Specific signs to watch for that indicate increasing risk
- When and how to contact you or other crisis team members
- Basic supportive responses that help vs. responses that might make things worse
- Documentation requirements for interactions with the student

Coping Strategies for School Hours

School-based coping strategies need to be portable, socially acceptable, and effective within the constraints of the educational environment.

Immediate coping strategies (use right now):

- Deep breathing techniques that can be done quietly in class

- Progressive muscle relaxation starting with hands and working up

- Grounding techniques using classroom objects (feel texture of desk, identify colors)

- Silent self-talk scripts ("this feeling will pass," "I am safe right now")

- Physical movement that's classroom-appropriate (stretching, foot exercises)

Short-term coping strategies (use during breaks):

- Walk to specific safe place in school (library, counselor's office, quiet hallway)

- Listen to specific calming music with headphones

- Write in journal or draw feelings

- Practice mindfulness exercises in bathroom or private space

- Connect with safe person for brief check-in

Class-based coping strategies:

- Request permission to step into hallway for 2-3 minutes

- Use agreed-upon signal to indicate need for support

- Focus on specific assignment or activity that provides distraction

- Practice breathing techniques that look like normal classroom behavior

- Use fidget tools or stress objects discretely

Between-class coping strategies:

- Quick check-in with safe staff member

- Brief visit to counselor's office or nurse

- Physical activity like walking stairs or going outside

- Connection with supportive peer

- Review safety plan reminders on phone

Emergency Contact Procedures

Every safety plan needs clear, specific procedures for getting help when coping strategies aren't working and suicidal thoughts become overwhelming.

School-based emergency procedures:

- Go immediately to nurse's office, counselor, or main office

- Ask any staff member to call specific safe person

- Use emergency signal or code word with safe staff members

- Call parent/guardian from school phone with staff support

- If unable to find safe person, go to main office and ask for help

After-school emergency procedures:

- Call parent/guardian immediately

- Contact crisis hotline if parents unavailable

- Go to emergency room if thoughts become overwhelming

- Contact mental health treatment provider if involved in care

- Use crisis text lines for immediate support

Weekend and holiday emergency procedures:

- Primary contact: parents/guardians with specific numbers

- Secondary contact: crisis hotlines and text lines

- Emergency services: 911 if immediate danger

- Mental health providers: after-hours numbers if available

- Trusted adult backup: specific family member or mentor

Technology-based support:

- Crisis text lines (text HOME to 741741)

- National Suicide Prevention Lifeline (988)

- Crisis apps with specific features student finds helpful

- Online support communities with appropriate oversight

- Video chat capabilities with family or professional supports when needed

The goal of school-based safety planning isn't to prevent all suicidal thoughts – it's to help students navigate those thoughts safely until the crisis passes and professional help can address underlying issues. Your safety plan becomes a bridge between the student's current crisis and their longer-term recovery and healing.

Chapter 3.2: Panic Attack Intervention

You hear rapid breathing coming from the supply closet near the gym. When you investigate, you find 14-year-old Emma hyperventilating, tears streaming down her face, clutching her chest. "I can't breathe," she gasps. "Something's wrong with my heart. I think I'm dying." Her lips are tinged blue, her hands are cramped into claws, and she's shaking uncontrollably. The PE teacher who found her is standing nearby, looking panicked himself.

This is a classic presentation of a panic attack, but in the moment, it can look like a serious medical emergency. Emma's symptoms are real – her body is having a genuine physiological response to perceived danger. But the "danger" exists in her mind, not in her environment. Your challenge is to quickly determine whether this is panic or something more serious, then intervene effectively to help her regain control of her nervous system.

Panic attacks are among the most dramatic mental health presentations you'll encounter in schools, but they're also among the most treatable. With the right interventions, you can usually help a student move from overwhelming terror to relative calm within 10-15 minutes. More importantly, students who learn to manage panic attacks often develop confidence and skills that serve them well beyond their school years.

Differential Diagnosis

The first and most critical step in panic attack intervention is determining whether you're dealing with panic or a genuine medical emergency. This differential diagnosis needs to happen quickly but thoroughly.

Medical vs. Panic Symptoms Checklist

Panic attacks mimic many serious medical conditions, which is part of what makes them so frightening for students experiencing them. However, certain patterns help distinguish panic from medical emergencies.

Symptoms that suggest panic attack:

- Rapid onset (symptoms peak within 10 minutes)

- Multiple symptoms happening simultaneously (racing heart, shortness of breath, sweating, trembling)

- Student can describe feeling terrified or having sense of impending doom

- Symptoms came on without obvious physical trigger

- Student has experienced similar episodes before

- Hyperventilation leading to tingling in hands/face

- No fever or other signs of illness

Red flags that suggest medical emergency:

- Chest pain that radiates to arm, jaw, or back

- Severe shortness of breath with wheezing or inability to speak

- High fever accompanying other symptoms

- Altered mental status (confusion, disorientation)

- Severe headache with visual changes

- Symptoms that started gradually and are getting progressively worse

- Student appears seriously ill rather than just terrified

- Abnormal vital signs beyond what's expected with anxiety

Key questions for differential diagnosis:

- "Have you felt like this before?" (panic attacks often recurrent)

- "Did this come on suddenly or gradually?" (panic is sudden onset)

- "Are you afraid something terrible is going to happen?" (classic panic cognition)

- "Can you tell me what you're feeling in your body right now?" (panic patients can usually describe symptoms clearly)

When to Call EMS

Certain presentations require emergency medical services, either because they represent genuine medical emergencies or because the student's symptoms are severe enough to require emergency evaluation.

Call 911 immediately for:

- Chest pain in student with known heart condition

- Severe breathing difficulty where student cannot speak in sentences

- Signs of heart attack (chest pain radiating to arm/jaw, sweating, nausea)

- Symptoms of stroke (facial drooping, arm weakness, speech problems)

- Altered mental status or loss of consciousness

- Severe allergic reaction signs

- Any situation where you're genuinely uncertain about medical vs. panic

Consider calling EMS for:

- First-time panic attack where student is convinced they're having medical emergency

- Panic attack that doesn't respond to usual interventions after 20-30 minutes

- Student with complex medical history where panic symptoms might mask other issues

- Family requests emergency evaluation

- Student becomes so distressed that you can't ensure their safety

Document decision-making: Always document your clinical reasoning about why you did or didn't call EMS. Include vital signs, specific symptoms observed, interventions attempted, and student response.

Cardiac Consideration Protocols

Since panic attacks often involve heart palpitations and chest sensations, you need specific protocols for evaluating cardiac symptoms.

When cardiac evaluation is warranted:

- Student reports chest pain as primary or severe symptom

- Heart rate over 150 bpm or under 50 bpm

- Irregular heart rhythm on pulse check

- Blood pressure significantly elevated (over 140/90 in teens)

- Student has known cardiac condition or family history of sudden cardiac death

- Chest pain that doesn't improve with panic interventions

Cardiac assessment steps:

1. Check pulse for rate, rhythm, and quality

2. Take blood pressure in both arms if possible

3. Ask about chest pain characteristics (sharp vs. pressure, location, radiation)

4. Listen to heart sounds if you're trained to do so

5. Check for peripheral pulses and skin color

6. Monitor oxygen saturation if pulse oximeter available

Documentation for cardiac concerns: Record exact vital signs, description of chest pain, timing of symptoms, and your clinical assessment. This information will be crucial if emergency services become involved.

Evidence-Based Interventions

Once you've determined that a student is experiencing a panic attack rather than a medical emergency, your interventions focus on helping them regain control of their nervous system and reducing the intensity of their symptoms.

TIPP Technique

TIPP stands for Temperature, Intense exercise, Paced breathing, and Paired muscle relaxation. This technique uses physiological principles to rapidly activate the parasympathetic nervous system and counteract panic symptoms.

T - Temperature: Use cold water or ice to activate the mammalian dive response, which naturally slows heart rate and reduces panic symptoms.

- Have student splash cold water on their face, particularly around eyes and upper cheeks

- Apply cold compress to forehead, temples, or back of neck

- Have them hold ice cubes in their hands

- Cold water bottle against pulse points (wrists, neck)

I - Intense Exercise: Brief, intense physical activity can metabolize stress hormones and redirect focus away from panic symptoms.

- 30 seconds of jumping jacks or running in place
- Push-ups against the wall (10-15 repetitions)
- Quick walk up and down stairs
- Rapid arm circles or other large muscle movements
- Only use if student is physically able and not too dizzy

P - Paced Breathing: Controlled breathing directly counteracts hyperventilation and helps regulate the autonomic nervous system.

- Box breathing: 4 counts in, 4 counts hold, 6 counts out, 4 counts hold
- Triangle breathing: 4 counts in, 4 counts hold, 6 counts out
- Paper bag breathing (only if available and student agrees)
- Focus on making exhale longer than inhale

P - Paired Muscle Relaxation: Progressive muscle relaxation helps release physical tension and provides concrete focus during panic.

- Start with hands: clench fists tight for 5 seconds, then release
- Move to arms: tense biceps, then release
- Shoulders: raise to ears, hold, then drop
- Face: scrunch all muscles, then relax
- Work systematically through major muscle groups

5-Minute Calming Protocol

When panic attacks occur, having a structured protocol helps ensure you don't forget important steps and gives both you and the student confidence that the situation is manageable.

Minutes 1-2: Assessment and rapport

- Move student to quiet, private space

- Introduce yourself calmly and assess immediate safety

- Validate their experience: "I can see this is really frightening"

- Begin teaching breathing: "Let's slow your breathing down together"

- Check vital signs if possible

Minutes 2-3: Active intervention

- Implement TIPP techniques based on what's most acceptable to student

- Guide breathing exercises consistently

- Provide constant reassurance: "You're safe, this will pass"

- Help them identify what they're experiencing in their body

- Continue calm, steady presence

Minutes 3-4: Stabilization

- Continue breathing exercises as symptoms begin to subside

- Help student identify that symptoms are decreasing

- Begin gentle grounding exercises (name 5 things you can see)

- Offer water or comfortable positioning

- Start exploring what triggered the attack

Minutes 4-5: Recovery planning

- Assess readiness to return to activities

- Discuss what helped and what didn't

- Plan for immediate follow-up and next steps

- Contact parents if appropriate
- Document the episode

Environmental Modifications

The physical environment can either help or hinder panic attack recovery. Simple modifications to your space and approach can significantly impact student outcomes.

Immediate environmental changes:

- Reduce stimulation: dim lights, minimize noise, clear clutter
- Provide comfortable seating or space to lie down
- Ensure privacy from other students and staff
- Remove crowds or audiences that might increase embarrassment
- Create calm atmosphere with your own demeanor and voice tone

Physical comfort measures:

- Offer blanket if student feels cold (common during panic)
- Provide tissues for tears or runny nose
- Ensure good ventilation without drafts
- Have water available (sips, not large amounts)
- Allow student to remove restrictive clothing (ties, tight collars)

Safety considerations:

- Position yourself between student and door (for your safety) without trapping them
- Remove any objects student might use to harm themselves in distress

- Ensure you can quickly get help if needed
- Be aware of student's physical position in case they faint

Post-Attack Procedures

What happens after the acute panic symptoms subside is crucial for the student's immediate wellbeing and their long-term relationship with panic attacks.

Recovery Time Guidelines

Students need adequate time to recover from panic attacks before returning to normal activities. Rushing this process can trigger another attack or create negative associations with school.

Physical recovery indicators:

- Heart rate returned to normal range (within 20 bpm of baseline)
- Breathing regular and unlabored
- No longer trembling or shaking
- Color returned to normal
- Able to hold conversation without breathlessness

Emotional recovery indicators:

- Student reports feeling calmer
- Able to talk about what happened without immediate re-triggering
- Expressing relief that symptoms are subsiding
- Showing some embarrassment or concern about missing class (indicates return to normal thinking)
- Able to problem-solve about next steps

Cognitive recovery indicators:

- Can focus on conversation with you
- Able to answer questions about their experience
- Demonstrates understanding that they had a panic attack
- Can participate in planning for return to activities
- Shows insight about possible triggers

Typical recovery timeline:

- Acute symptoms: 5-20 minutes
- Physical recovery: 30-60 minutes
- Full emotional recovery: 1-3 hours
- Some fatigue may persist for several hours

Return-to-Class Readiness Assessment

Determining when a student is ready to return to class requires assessment of multiple factors beyond just symptom resolution.

Readiness checklist:

- Physical symptoms completely resolved
- Student expresses readiness to return (not just compliance with your suggestion)
- Has plan for what to do if symptoms return
- Understands they can come back to you if needed
- Able to focus on something other than the panic attack
- Not worried about immediate recurrence

Modifications for initial return:

- Shortened class periods initially
- Permission to leave class if symptoms return

- Modified participation in physical activities
- Extra time for assignments due that day
- Check-in plan with teacher or other safe person

When to delay return:

- Student expresses fear about returning to triggering situation
- Physical symptoms haven't completely resolved
- Multiple panic attacks in same day
- Student seems disconnected or "spacey"
- Triggering situation (test, presentation) hasn't been addressed

Prevention Planning for Future Attacks

Students who have experienced panic attacks are at higher risk for future episodes, but they're also in a prime position to learn prevention and management strategies.

Immediate prevention planning:

- Identify triggers from this episode
- Discuss early warning signs student noticed
- Practice breathing techniques while calm
- Plan for what to do if symptoms start to return
- Identify safe spaces and people at school

Trigger identification:

- What was happening right before the attack?
- What thoughts were going through their mind?
- Any physical sensations they noticed first?

- Environmental factors (crowded space, test situation, conflict)?

- Timing patterns (certain times of day, days of week)?

Early warning sign recognition:

- First physical sensations they remember

- Changes in thinking or worry patterns

- Environmental situations that make them nervous

- Physical signs others might notice (fidgeting, avoiding eye contact)

- Behavioral changes that precede attacks

Coping strategy development:

- Which TIPP techniques worked best for them?

- Breathing exercises they found most helpful

- Environmental modifications they prefer

- People they feel comfortable approaching for help

- Self-talk strategies that help them stay calm

Teacher Notification Templates

Teachers need to understand how to support students returning from panic attacks without creating embarrassment or drawing unwanted attention.

Basic teacher notification: "Sarah is returning to class after experiencing some anxiety. She's feeling better now but might need a few minutes to settle back in. Please check in with her quietly in about 15 minutes to see how she's doing."

For students with recurrent panic attacks: "David sometimes experiences panic attacks and has learned some good coping strategies. If you notice him looking anxious or asking to step into the hallway, please let him do so and send him to me if he requests it. These episodes are medical in nature and he's learning to manage them well."

For teachers who witnessed the panic attack: "Emma experienced a panic attack earlier, which can look very scary but isn't dangerous. She's learned some breathing techniques and knows to come to me if she needs help. Panic attacks are common and treatable - she's getting good support and learning to manage them."

Specific accommodation requests: "For the next few days, Alex might need permission to step out of class briefly if they're feeling anxious. This is part of their treatment plan for managing panic attacks. Please don't make a big deal of it, just let them know they can step into the hall or come see me if needed."

Chapter 3.3: Aggressive Behavior Response

The sound of shouting draws you toward the math hallway. As you round the corner, you see 15-year-old Marcus standing face-to-face with his teacher, fists clenched, face red with anger. "You can't make me!" he's yelling. "I'm not doing your stupid assignment!" Other students have backed away, some looking scared, others pulling out phones to record the confrontation. The teacher looks uncertain whether to approach or retreat.

Aggressive behavior in schools creates immediate safety concerns for everyone involved – the aggressive student, their peers, staff members, and bystanders. But underneath that anger and aggression is almost always a young person who feels overwhelmed, misunderstood, or backed into a corner. Your response in these moments can either escalate the situation into something dangerous or help the student regain control and find more appropriate ways to express their distress.

The key to effective aggressive behavior response is understanding that aggression is usually a symptom of underlying distress rather than just "bad behavior." Students don't typically want to be aggressive – they want to be heard, respected, and understood. When those needs aren't met through appropriate channels, aggression becomes their way of communicating that something is seriously wrong.

De-escalation Hierarchy

De-escalation is both an art and a science. It requires you to remain calm under pressure, accurately read the student's emotional state, and respond in ways that reduce rather than increase their distress. The hierarchy approach gives you a systematic way to try different interventions, starting with the least intrusive and moving toward more intensive responses as needed.

Verbal De-escalation Techniques

Your words, tone, and timing can be the difference between a situation that resolves peacefully and one that escalates into physical confrontation or emergency response.

Level 1 - Supportive listening:

- "I can see you're really upset about something"
- "Help me understand what's happening for you right now"
- "It sounds like this situation is really frustrating"
- "Tell me what's going on from your perspective"

Level 2 - Validation and empathy:

- "That does sound really frustrating"
- "I can understand why you'd be angry about that"
- "It makes sense that you'd be upset"
- "Your feelings are valid, even though we need to find a better way to handle this"

Level 3 - Collaborative problem-solving:

- "Let's figure out how to solve this together"
- "What would help make this situation better?"
- "What do you need right now to feel calmer?"
- "How can we work this out in a way that feels fair to everyone?"

Level 4 - Clear boundaries with choices:

- "I need you to lower your voice so we can work this out"
- "You can choose to talk with me here, or we can go somewhere more private"

- "Right now you need to step away from [the situation/person] so we can calm down"
- "Help me help you by taking some deep breaths with me"

Verbal techniques to avoid:

- Commands or demands ("Calm down right now!")
- Threats or ultimatums ("If you don't stop, you'll be suspended")
- Dismissive language ("You're overreacting")
- Logic arguments when emotions are high ("That doesn't make sense")
- Comparisons to other students ("Other kids don't act this way")

Body Language and Positioning

Your physical presence communicates as much as your words. Students who are already agitated are hypervigilant to signs of threat, so your body language needs to communicate safety and calm.

Calming body language:

- Keep hands visible and open (not crossed or behind back)
- Stand at slight angle rather than directly facing (less threatening)
- Maintain comfortable distance (arm's length plus a few feet)
- Keep your posture relaxed but alert
- Make eye contact but don't stare
- Move slowly and deliberately

Positioning for safety and effectiveness:

- Position yourself between the student and potential triggers (other students, confrontational adults)

- Stay close to exit routes for both you and the student

- Avoid cornering or trapping the student

- Be aware of objects that could become weapons if grabbed

- Position yourself where you can signal for help if needed

What your body language should convey:

- "I'm here to help, not to punish"

- "I'm not afraid of you, but I respect that you're upset"

- "I'm confident we can work this out"

- "You're safe with me"

- "I have time for you"

When to Call for Backup

Knowing when to call for additional help is crucial for everyone's safety. Calling too early might escalate the situation, but waiting too long could put people at risk.

Call for backup immediately when:

- Student threatens physical violence toward anyone

- Student picks up or reaches for potential weapons

- Student's agitation is increasing despite de-escalation attempts

- Multiple students are becoming involved or agitated

- You feel genuinely unsafe or threatened

- Student is destroying property in ways that could cause injury

- Situation is drawing crowds that might escalate things

Consider calling backup when:

- De-escalation attempts aren't showing progress after 10-15 minutes

- Student has history of physical aggression

- You're feeling overwhelmed or unsure how to proceed

- Situation involves multiple complex issues requiring team response

- Student is requesting specific person who might be more effective

How to call for backup effectively:

- Use predetermined signals or code words when possible

- Specify type of help needed (administrator, counselor, security, police)

- Provide brief, factual description of situation

- Indicate urgency level

- Continue de-escalation while waiting for help to arrive

CPI Principles Adaptation

Crisis Prevention Institute (CPI) principles provide evidence-based approaches for managing behavioral crises. These can be adapted for school nursing contexts.

Supportive stance:

- Non-threatening posture with hands at sides

- Respectful interpersonal distance

- Calm, low voice tone

- Non-confrontational facial expression

Empathic listening:

- Focus on understanding student's perspective
- Reflect back what you're hearing
- Validate emotions while addressing behaviors
- Ask open-ended questions to understand underlying needs

Rational detachment:

- Don't take aggressive behavior personally
- Maintain professional composure even when student is hostile
- Focus on helping rather than winning or being right
- Stay objective about what's happening and why

Integrated experience:

- Consider the whole person, not just the problematic behavior
- Understand that aggression usually indicates pain or distress
- Look for underlying needs driving the aggressive behavior
- Respond to the person behind the behavior

Safety First Protocols

When aggressive behavior occurs, ensuring everyone's physical safety takes precedence over all other concerns, including therapeutic relationships and educational goals.

Clearing the Area Procedures

Removing audiences and potential targets reduces both safety risks and embarrassment for the aggressive student.

Immediate area clearing:

- Direct other students to move to specific safe location

- Give clear, calm instructions: "Everyone please move to the other side of the hallway"
- Don't shout or sound panicked (this escalates everyone's anxiety)
- Ask specific students to help guide others away
- Close doors to classrooms if possible to contain situation

Crowd management:

- Prevent students from recording with phones or gathering to watch
- Ask teachers to keep their students in classrooms
- Clear a wide perimeter around the aggressive student
- Ensure exit routes remain available for everyone
- Designate specific person to manage crowd if backup arrives

Protecting vulnerable individuals:

- Move younger students away first
- Ensure students with disabilities or anxiety don't get overlooked
- Check that no one is trapped or cornered
- Account for all students who were initially in the area
- Provide reassurance to witnesses that they're safe

Staff Communication Systems

Effective communication during aggressive behavior incidents ensures appropriate response and prevents confusion or conflicting interventions.

Initial communication:

- Alert main office immediately about location and nature of incident

- Request specific types of backup needed

- Inform administrators about students involved

- Update other nearby staff about situation status

Ongoing communication:

- Provide brief updates if situation changes significantly

- Alert when situation is resolved or when emergency services needed

- Communicate if incident is moving to different location

- Update about injuries or property damage

Post-incident communication:

- Debrief with all staff who were involved

- Share lessons learned and what worked well

- Discuss any changes needed to protocols

- Ensure all required notifications have been made

Documentation of Incidents

Thorough documentation of aggressive behavior incidents is essential for legal protection, pattern identification, and continuous improvement of response protocols.

Document immediately while fresh in memory:

- Exact time and location of incident

- Names of all individuals involved and witnesses

- Sequence of events leading up to aggressive behavior

- Specific behaviors observed (threats, physical actions, property damage)

- Exact words spoken by all parties when possible

- De-escalation techniques attempted and student responses

- When and what type of backup was called

- How situation was resolved

- Any injuries or property damage

- Follow-up actions taken

Objective vs. subjective documentation:

- *Objective:* "Student threw textbook across room, hitting wall"

- *Subjective:* "Student was out of control and furious"

- *Objective:* "Student said 'I'm going to punch someone if you don't leave me alone'"

- *Subjective:* "Student threatened everyone in the room"

Post-Incident Procedures

How you handle the aftermath of aggressive behavior incidents significantly impacts the student's future behavior, peer relationships, and overall school climate.

Medical Assessment for Injuries

Even minor aggressive incidents can result in injuries that need attention, and sometimes injuries aren't immediately apparent due to adrenaline.

Check all involved parties:

- Aggressive student (may have injured themselves)

- Anyone who was target of aggression

- Bystanders who may have been accidentally hurt
- Staff members who intervened

Types of injuries to assess:

- Obvious injuries from hitting or throwing objects
- Strain or sprain injuries from physical restraint
- Scratches or bruises from grabbing or pushing
- Stress-related symptoms in witnesses (headaches, nausea)
- Emotional trauma responses that manifest physically

Documentation of injuries:

- Photograph injuries if appropriate and with consent
- Describe location, size, and appearance of any marks
- Note student's report of pain or discomfort
- Record any first aid provided
- Determine if additional medical evaluation needed

Emotional Support for Involved Students

Aggressive incidents are traumatic for everyone involved, including the student who was aggressive. Each person needs different types of support.

Supporting the aggressive student:

- Process what happened without judgment
- Help them understand the impact of their behavior
- Explore underlying triggers and needs
- Develop alternative coping strategies
- Plan for prevention of future incidents

- Address any shame or embarrassment they're feeling

Supporting target students:

- Validate that the experience was frightening

- Ensure they understand it wasn't their fault

- Address any self-blame or wondering what they did wrong

- Provide safety planning for future interactions

- Consider counseling referral if trauma symptoms develop

- Help them process their emotions about the incident

Supporting witness students:

- Acknowledge that witnessing aggression can be scary

- Answer questions they have about what happened

- Normalize their emotional reactions

- Provide reassurance about their safety at school

- Watch for signs of ongoing anxiety or trauma

- Consider classroom discussion about handling conflicts

Witness Support Protocols

Students who witness aggressive behavior need support to process what they've seen and maintain their sense of safety at school.

Immediate witness support:

- Move witnesses to safe, calm environment

- Do quick check-in about how they're feeling

- Provide factual information about what will happen next

- Avoid detailed discussion of the incident immediately

- Connect them with counselors or safe adults as needed

149

Follow-up witness support:

- Individual check-ins with students who seemed most affected
- Classroom discussion about conflict resolution and safety
- Teaching about when and how to get adult help
- Reinforcing that they did the right thing by staying safe
- Ongoing monitoring for signs of anxiety or trauma

Parent communication about witness trauma:

- Inform parents that their child witnessed concerning incident
- Describe what support was provided at school
- Give guidance about signs of trauma to watch for at home
- Provide resources for additional support if needed
- Maintain confidentiality about details of incident

Threat Assessment Procedures

Not all aggressive behavior represents ongoing threat, but systematic assessment helps determine appropriate response and prevention strategies.

Immediate threat assessment questions:

- Does student continue to express intent to harm others?
- Do they have access to weapons or means to cause significant harm?
- Are there specific targets they've identified?
- Is there evidence of planning for future aggressive acts?
- Do they show remorse or understanding of impact of their behavior?

Factors that increase ongoing threat:

- History of escalating aggressive behavior

- Access to weapons at home or school

- Social isolation or rejection by peer groups

- Recent significant losses or traumas

- Substance use or mental health issues

- Exposure to violence or aggressive role models

Factors that decrease ongoing threat:

- Student expresses genuine remorse for behavior

- Incident was clearly triggered by specific, resolvable situation

- Student has good support system and protective relationships

- Previous aggressive incidents were rare and situational

- Student is willing to engage in help and behavior planning

Re-entry Planning

Getting students back to normal school routines after aggressive incidents requires careful planning that addresses safety, relationships, and learning.

Behavior Plan Coordination

Effective behavior planning involves the student, family, and school team working together to prevent future incidents and support positive behavior.

Behavior plan components:

- Clear identification of triggers that lead to aggressive behavior

- Alternative coping strategies for managing frustration and anger

- Environmental modifications to reduce likelihood of triggers

- Positive reinforcement for appropriate behavior and conflict resolution

- Clear consequences for future aggressive behavior

- Regular check-ins and plan adjustments as needed

Team members to involve:

- Student (as primary participant in plan development)

- Parents or guardians

- School administrators

- Teachers who work with the student regularly

- School counselor or social worker

- Special education staff if applicable

Medication Considerations

Some students who display aggressive behavior are taking medications that might be contributing factors, while others might benefit from medication evaluation.

Medication review considerations:

- Side effects of current medications that might increase irritability

- Timing of medication doses and relationship to aggressive incidents

- Recent changes in medications or dosages

- Need for medication evaluation if behavior represents new pattern

- Coordination with healthcare providers about behavior observations

School-based medication monitoring:

- Document behavior patterns in relation to medication timing
- Watch for side effects that might affect mood or behavior
- Communicate with parents and healthcare providers about observations
- Ensure medication compliance isn't contributing to behavior issues

Support Team Assembly

Students with aggressive behavior need comprehensive support teams that address underlying causes while maintaining safety and accountability.

Core team members:

- School nurse (medical and crisis response perspective)
- School counselor (emotional and behavioral support)
- Administrator (discipline and safety oversight)
- Teacher representatives (academic and classroom management perspective)
- Parents/guardians (home context and family dynamics)

Extended team members when appropriate:

- Special education staff if disabilities are involved
- Mental health professionals treating the student
- Community mentors or support persons
- Peer mediators for relationship repair
- Law enforcement if legal issues are involved

Your Crisis Response Toolkit

You now have detailed protocols for managing the three most challenging crisis situations you'll face: suicidal ideation, panic attacks, and aggressive behavior. Each requires different skills and different immediate responses, but they share common elements: the need for calm, systematic intervention that prioritizes safety while preserving dignity and therapeutic relationships.

Your crisis response skills will improve with practice and experience, but having solid protocols gives you confidence to act decisively when students need help most. The practical tools included with this section – crisis response flip cards, emergency contact sheets, incident documentation forms, and de-escalation technique reminders – will help you implement these protocols effectively.

Most importantly, you're not expected to handle these crises alone. Your role is to provide immediate stabilization and connect students with appropriate longer-term support. These protocols help you do that job safely and effectively while maintaining your own wellbeing and professional boundaries.

The investment you make in mastering crisis response protocols pays dividends not just in emergency situations, but in building a school environment where students feel safe, supported, and confident that caring adults will help them through their most difficult moments.

Section 4: Communication Scripts

Chapter 4.1: Talking to Students

The words you choose in those first moments when a student sits down across from you can set the entire tone for what follows. Sixteen-year-old Taylor shuffles into your office, avoiding eye contact, shoulders hunched defensively. They were sent by their English teacher who noticed concerning changes in their behavior over the past few weeks. How you open this conversation will determine whether Taylor opens up about what's really happening or shuts down completely.

Communication with students about mental health isn't just about gathering information – it's about creating a space where young people feel safe enough to share their most vulnerable thoughts and feelings. Students are experts at reading adults. They can sense within seconds whether you're genuinely interested in understanding them or just going through the motions of asking required questions.

Your communication skills as a school nurse dealing with mental health concerns require a different approach than your medical nursing communication. When you're treating a physical injury, students generally want you to fix the problem quickly and efficiently. But when you're addressing emotional distress, students need to feel heard, understood, and respected as the experts on their own experiences.

Building Rapport Quickly

Rapport isn't something that happens automatically because you're a caring person or because you have good intentions. It's a skill that requires intentional choices about your words, your body language, and your approach to each individual student.

Age-Appropriate Opening Statements

Different age groups respond to different communication styles, and what builds rapport with a 7-year-old will likely feel patronizing to a 17-year-old.

Elementary students (ages 5-11):

- "Hi there! I'm Mrs. Johnson, the school nurse. I heard you might be having a tough day today."

- "Your teacher told me you've been feeling sad lately. Can you tell me about that?"

- "I know sometimes big feelings can make your tummy hurt or give you headaches. Is that happening with you?"

- "It takes courage to come talk to an adult when you're feeling upset. I'm really glad you're here."

Elementary students respond to warm, nurturing language that acknowledges their emotions while using vocabulary they understand. They appreciate when adults recognize their bravery in seeking help.

Middle school students (ages 11-14):

- "Thanks for coming to see me. I know this might feel awkward, but I'm here to listen to whatever is going on with you."

- "Your counselor mentioned you've been struggling with some things. I'm wondering how I can help."

- "Sometimes middle school can be really tough. What's been the hardest part for you lately?"

- "I meet with lots of students who are dealing with stress and difficult feelings. You're definitely not alone in this."

157

Middle schoolers are beginning to develop adult-like thinking but still need reassurance that their problems are normal and that adults take them seriously.

High school students (ages 14-18):

- "I appreciate you taking time to meet with me. What's been going on that brought you here today?"

- "I'm hearing from several people that you've been having a difficult time lately. Help me understand your perspective."

- "Mental health is just as important as physical health, and I treat both with equal seriousness. What's going on for you right now?"

- "You know yourself better than anyone else. I'm hoping you can help me understand what you're experiencing."

Older teens want to be treated as capable young adults who have valuable insights about their own experiences. They respond well to direct, respectful communication that doesn't talk down to them.

Creating Psychological Safety

Psychological safety means students feel they can be honest without fear of judgment, punishment, or unwanted consequences. Creating this safety requires both your words and your overall approach.

Verbal strategies for psychological safety:

- Use "I" statements: "I'm concerned about you" rather than "You have a problem"

- Ask open-ended questions: "What's been going on for you?" rather than "Are you depressed?"

- Validate their experience: "That sounds really difficult" before moving to problem-solving

- Normalize struggle: "Many students go through tough times" helps reduce shame

- Express genuine curiosity: "Help me understand" communicates that you want to learn from them

Non-verbal strategies for psychological safety:

- Sit at their eye level rather than standing over them

- Keep your body language open (uncrossed arms, relaxed posture)

- Make eye contact but don't stare intensely

- Match their energy level (if they're speaking softly, you speak softly too)

- Remove physical barriers like desks between you when possible

Environmental strategies:

- Meet in a private space where they won't be overheard or interrupted

- Turn off or silence phones and computers to show you're fully present

- Have tissues available and other comfort items

- Ensure the space feels welcoming rather than clinical

- Position chairs so they can easily leave if they need to

Confidentiality Explanations with Limits

Students need to understand both what you will keep private and what you're required to share with others. Being upfront about confidentiality limits actually builds trust rather than damaging it.

How to explain confidentiality to students: "I want you to feel comfortable talking with me, so let me explain how confidentiality works. Most of what you tell me stays between us. I don't share information with your parents, teachers, or friends without your permission. But there are a few situations where I have to involve other adults to keep you safe..."

The limits you must explain:

- "If you tell me someone is hurting you or you're in danger, I need to get help"

- "If you're thinking about hurting yourself or someone else, I need to involve other people to keep everyone safe"

- "If you're being hurt by an adult, I'm required by law to report that"

- "Sometimes I might need to work with other school staff to help you, but I'll talk with you about that first"

Age-appropriate confidentiality explanations:

Elementary: "I keep secrets that are safe secrets, but if someone is hurting you or you might get hurt, I need to tell other grown-ups who can help keep you safe."

Middle school: "I won't tell your parents or teachers what we talk about unless you want me to, but if you're not safe or someone is hurting you, I have to get other adults involved to help protect you."

High school: "Our conversations are confidential, which means private between us, except in situations where safety is a concern. If you're thinking about suicide, being abused, or planning to hurt someone, I'm required to involve other people. But I'll always try to involve you in deciding how to handle those situations."

Therapeutic Communication Techniques

Therapeutic communication goes beyond just being nice or supportive. It involves specific techniques designed to help students explore their feelings, gain insight into their experiences, and feel genuinely understood.

Active Listening Demonstrations

Active listening is more than just hearing words – it's about understanding the meaning behind what students are saying and communicating that understanding back to them.

Components of active listening:

Full attention: Put away distractions, face the student, and focus completely on what they're saying. Students can tell when you're multitasking or thinking about other things.

Reflective listening: Repeat back what you're hearing in your own words. "It sounds like you're saying that even though you're doing well in school, you feel really sad most of the time."

Emotional reflection: Identify and reflect the emotions you're hearing. "You seem frustrated that nobody seems to understand how hard things are for you right now."

Clarifying questions: Ask questions that help you understand better. "When you say you feel 'weird,' can you help me understand what that feels like in your body?"

Summarizing: Periodically pull together what you've heard. "Let me make sure I understand. You've been feeling really anxious about tests, you're not sleeping well, and your friends have been commenting that you seem different."

Examples of active listening in action:

Student says: "I don't know why everyone thinks there's something wrong with me. I'm fine."

Poor response: "But your teacher is worried about you."

Active listening response: "It sounds like you're frustrated that people are concerned about you when you feel like you're managing okay. Help me understand your perspective on how things are going."

Student says: "My parents are getting divorced and it's all my fault."

Poor response: "I'm sure it's not your fault."

Active listening response: "That must be an incredibly heavy feeling, thinking that you caused your parents' problems. Can you tell me more about why you think you're responsible?"

Validation Without Agreement

Validation means acknowledging that a student's feelings make sense given their experience, even if you don't agree with their interpretation of events or their planned actions.

What validation sounds like:

- "That sounds incredibly frustrating"

- "I can understand why you'd feel angry about that"

- "It makes sense that you'd be worried given what's been happening"

- "Your feelings are completely understandable"

- "Anyone in your situation would probably feel overwhelmed"

What validation is NOT:

- Agreeing with factually incorrect statements

- Endorsing harmful plans or behaviors

- Taking sides in conflicts

- Minimizing the complexity of situations

- Avoiding necessary limit-setting or safety measures

Examples of validation without agreement:

Student: "I'm stupid and worthless. I should just kill myself." *Validation:* "It sounds like you're in tremendous emotional pain right now, and dying feels like the only way to make it stop. Those feelings must be overwhelming." *Without agreement:* You're validating their

162

pain without agreeing that they're worthless or that suicide is a good solution.

Student: "My teacher hates me and is trying to fail me on purpose." *Validation:* "It must feel really discouraging to think your teacher is against you. That would make school feel pretty hopeless." *Without agreement:* You're validating their discouragement without agreeing that the teacher actually hates them.

Motivational Interviewing Basics

Motivational interviewing is a counseling approach that helps people explore their ambivalence about change and find their own motivation for making positive choices.

Key principles of motivational interviewing:

Express empathy: Try to understand the student's perspective without judgment.

Develop discrepancy: Help students see the gap between their current situation and their goals or values.

Roll with resistance: Don't argue with students who are reluctant to change. Instead, explore their resistance.

Support self-efficacy: Express confidence in the student's ability to make positive changes.

Motivational interviewing techniques for school nurses:

Open-ended questions: "What concerns you most about your current situation?" rather than "Are you worried about your grades?"

Affirmations: "It took courage to come talk to me about this" or "You've shown real strength in dealing with this situation."

Reflections: "You're torn between wanting to feel better and not wanting to deal with the work that therapy might involve."

Summaries: "On one hand, you're exhausted by feeling anxious all the time. On the other hand, you're worried that getting help might make things more complicated."

Difficult Conversation Scripts

Some conversations are inherently difficult, but having prepared scripts helps you navigate these challenging discussions with confidence and skill.

"I'm Worried About You Because..."

This phrase is powerful because it expresses care while being specific about your concerns. Students respond better to concrete observations than to vague expressions of worry.

Effective "worried about you" statements:

- "I'm worried about you because I've noticed you've been coming to the nurse's office almost every day this month, and you seem really distressed each time."

- "I'm worried about you because your grades have dropped significantly, and several teachers have mentioned that you seem withdrawn in class."

- "I'm worried about you because you mentioned having trouble sleeping and not enjoying things you used to love, which can be signs that you're struggling with depression."

- "I'm worried about you because you've been losing weight rapidly, and I've noticed you avoiding the cafeteria during lunch."

Why this approach works:

- It expresses genuine care rather than criticism

- It provides specific, observable reasons for concern

- It opens the door for the student to share more information

- It positions you as an ally rather than an adversary

Discussing Self-Harm Discoveries

When you discover that a student has been engaging in self-harm behaviors, your initial response sets the tone for their willingness to engage in safety planning and seek help.

Initial response scripts: "I noticed some cuts on your arm, and I'm concerned about you. Can you help me understand what's been going on that led to this?"

"Your friend came to me because they're worried about you hurting yourself. I can see this might feel like a betrayal, but they care about you and so do I. Can we talk about what's happening?"

"I see some marks that look like they might be from hurting yourself. I'm not angry or disappointed – I'm concerned and want to understand how you've been feeling."

What NOT to say:

- "Why would you do this to yourself?" (implies judgment)
- "This isn't going to solve your problems" (dismissive)
- "How could you hurt yourself like this?" (expresses shock and horror)
- "Promise me you won't do this again" (creates pressure for unrealistic promises)

Follow-up conversation elements:

- Explore the function self-harm serves for them
- Discuss alternative coping strategies
- Address safety concerns without being controlling
- Involve appropriate support people
- Develop safety planning collaboratively

Addressing Substance Use Concerns

Students are often defensive about substance use because they fear punishment, lectures, or loss of autonomy. Your approach needs to be curious and non-judgmental.

Opening scripts for substance use discussions: "I've noticed some signs that make me wonder if you might be using alcohol or drugs to cope with stress. I'm not here to get you in trouble – I'm concerned about your health and wellbeing."

"Several people have mentioned that they're worried you might be using substances. Rather than me guessing what's going on, can you help me understand your experience?"

"Lots of teenagers experiment with alcohol and drugs, especially when they're dealing with difficult emotions. I'm wondering if that's something you've been trying."

Exploratory questions:

- "What substances have you tried, and how often are you using them?"

- "How do you feel before you use, and how do you feel afterward?"

- "What role does substance use play in helping you cope with stress?"

- "Have you noticed any negative effects from your substance use?"

- "What concerns, if any, do you have about your substance use?"

LGBTQ+ Affirming Language

LGBTQ+ students experience mental health challenges at significantly higher rates than their peers, with 65% reporting persistent sadness. Your language can either increase their sense of safety or inadvertently cause harm.

Affirming language strategies:

- Use gender-neutral language initially: "Are you interested in dating anyone?" rather than assuming heterosexuality

- Ask about pronouns: "What pronouns do you use?" or "How would you like me to refer to you?"

- Use inclusive relationship terms: "partner," "significant other," or "person you're dating"

- Avoid assumptions about family structure: "the adults who take care of you" rather than assuming traditional parents

Specific affirming phrases:

- "Thank you for trusting me with this information about your identity"

- "I want to make sure I'm using the right name and pronouns for you"

- "Your identity is valid, and you deserve to feel safe and supported"

- "Some families need time to understand and accept their child's identity – that's not a reflection on you"

- "There are resources and communities where you can connect with other LGBTQ+ young people"

Addressing specific LGBTQ+ mental health concerns:

- Minority stress and its impact on mental health

- Family rejection or lack of acceptance

- Bullying or harassment related to identity

- Lack of representation or role models

- Concerns about safety and disclosure

Cultural Competency Considerations

Students from different cultural backgrounds may have very different relationships with mental health, help-seeking, and authority figures. Effective communication requires understanding and adapting to these differences.

Language Barriers and Interpreter Use

When students have limited English proficiency, you need strategies that ensure accurate communication while maintaining confidentiality and rapport.

Best practices for working with interpreters:

- Use trained medical interpreters when possible, not family members

- Speak directly to the student, not the interpreter

- Use first person: "I feel sad" not "She says she feels sad"

- Pause frequently to allow for interpretation

- Be aware that some concepts don't translate directly across languages

- Ask the interpreter to use the exact words when possible, not to summarize

Working without interpreters:

- Speak slowly and clearly, but don't talk louder

- Use simple vocabulary and avoid idioms

- Use visual aids, gestures, and written materials when helpful

- Check for understanding frequently

- Be patient with processing time

- Consider using translation apps as supplementary tools, not primary communication

Cultural considerations in mental health terminology:

- Some cultures don't have direct equivalents for terms like "depression" or "anxiety"
- Mental health symptoms might be expressed through physical complaints
- Some cultures view mental health problems as spiritual or moral issues
- Stigma around mental health varies significantly across cultures

Cultural Stigma Navigation

Different cultures have varying levels of stigma around mental health, and some families may view seeking help as shameful or dangerous.

Common cultural barriers to mental health help-seeking:

- Belief that mental health problems reflect personal weakness or moral failing
- Fear that mental health diagnosis will bring shame to the entire family
- Religious beliefs that attribute mental health problems to spiritual causes
- Mistrust of authority figures or government systems
- Previous negative experiences with mental health services
- Economic concerns about cost of treatment

Strategies for addressing cultural stigma:

- Acknowledge that you understand seeking help can be difficult in some cultures

- Frame mental health in terms of overall wellness and functioning
- Emphasize confidentiality and privacy protections
- Connect families with culturally competent mental health providers
- Use community liaisons or cultural brokers when available
- Provide education about mental health in culturally appropriate ways

Family Structure Variations

Families come in many different configurations, and your communication needs to account for these variations without making assumptions.

Avoiding assumptions about family structure:

- Don't assume students live with biological parents
- Use terms like "the adults who take care of you" or "your family"
- Ask who should be contacted in emergencies rather than assuming
- Understand that decision-making authority may not rest with legal guardians
- Be aware that some families have complex custody or immigration situations

Common family structures to be aware of:

- Single-parent households
- Grandparents or other relatives as primary caregivers
- Blended families with step-parents and step-siblings

- Families with same-sex parents
- Multigenerational households with multiple decision-makers
- Foster families or kinship care arrangements
- Families where parents work multiple jobs or travel frequently

Communication adaptations for different family structures:

- Ask about family dynamics and who makes decisions about healthcare
- Understand that some students may be caring for younger siblings or elderly relatives
- Be sensitive to economic pressures that might affect treatment decisions
- Recognize that family support systems may look different than traditional models
- Adapt your recommendations to fit the family's actual structure and resources

Chapter 4.2: Parent Communication Strategies

The phone call you're about to make will change everything for this family. Maria's parents think their 15-year-old daughter is just going through typical teenage moodiness, but you've just completed a screening that suggests she's experiencing significant depression with some suicidal thoughts. How you deliver this information will determine whether the family becomes a partner in Maria's recovery or reacts with denial, anger, or panic that makes the situation worse.

Parent communication about mental health requires a different skill set than almost any other conversation you'll have as a school nurse. Parents are often caught completely off guard by mental health concerns. They may feel guilty, defensive, overwhelmed, or frightened. Their initial reaction might be to minimize the problem, blame the school, or panic about what this means for their child's future.

Your job is to navigate these complex emotions while ensuring that parents have the information and support they need to help their child. This means being clear and direct about concerning symptoms while also being compassionate about the family's experience and realistic about next steps.

Initial Contact Protocols

The way you initiate contact with parents about mental health concerns sets the tone for your entire ongoing relationship around their child's wellbeing.

Phone vs. In-Person Decisions

The urgency and complexity of the situation help determine whether to use phone contact or request an in-person meeting.

Use phone contact for:

- Immediate safety concerns that require same-day parent involvement

- Initial notification about moderate mental health concerns

- Routine updates about ongoing mental health support

- Quick consultation about medication side effects or appointment scheduling

- Situations where parents have specifically requested phone contact

Request in-person meetings for:

- Complex mental health situations requiring detailed discussion

- When delivering concerning assessment results that need explanation

- Situations involving multiple school staff or treatment providers

- When parents have expressed confusion or resistance over the phone

- Developing comprehensive support plans or safety plans

- Initial meetings with parents who are new to mental health concerns

Consider virtual meetings for:

- Parents who have difficulty coming to school due to work schedules

- Situations where multiple family members need to participate

- Follow-up meetings that don't require in-person presence

- Families who prefer technology-mediated communication

Opening Statement Templates

Your opening words need to communicate concern while avoiding panic, provide enough information to explain why you're calling, and set a collaborative rather than confrontational tone.

For urgent concerns: "Hello, Mrs. Rodriguez. This is Sarah Johnson, the school nurse at Lincoln High School. I'm calling about Maria because I have some immediate concerns about her safety and wellbeing. She's safe right now and here with me, but I need to talk with you about what's happening and what we need to do next."

For significant but non-urgent concerns: "Hi, Mr. Kim. This is calling from school about Alex. I wanted to talk with you about some mental health concerns that have come up during our routine screening. Alex isn't in any immediate danger, but I think it's important for us to discuss what I'm observing and what might be helpful for them."

For ongoing support coordination: "Good afternoon, Mrs. Johnson. I'm calling to update you on how David has been doing with the mental health support we put in place last month, and to see how things are going at home."

For routine prevention/education: "Hello, this is from the school. I'm calling to let you know about our mental health screening program and to answer any questions you might have about what this involves for Emma."

Information Organization Strategies

Before making difficult phone calls, organize your information in a way that helps you communicate clearly and respond to parents' likely questions.

Information to have ready:

- Specific observations that led to your concern
- Results of any screening tools or assessments completed

- Timeline of when you first noticed concerning signs

- Current safety measures in place

- Specific recommendations for next steps

- Names and contact information for local mental health resources

- Your availability for follow-up questions or meetings

Organize information by priority:

1. Most important information (safety concerns, urgent recommendations)

2. Supporting details (specific symptoms, assessment results)

3. Resources and next steps

4. Answers to common questions

Anticipate common parent questions:

- "How long has this been going on?"

- "Why didn't anyone tell us sooner?"

- "Is this something we caused?"

- "What does this mean for their future?"

- "How much will treatment cost?"

- "Can't we just handle this ourselves?"

Delivering Difficult News

When you need to tell parents that their child is struggling with mental health concerns, your approach can either facilitate acceptance and action or create resistance and denial.

Suicide Risk Notification Script

This is perhaps the most difficult conversation you'll ever have with parents, and it requires careful balance between urgency and calm.

Script framework: "Mr. and Mrs. Thompson, I need to talk with you about some very serious concerns about Jake's safety. During a mental health screening today, he told me that he's been having thoughts about not wanting to be alive and has been thinking about ways he might hurt himself. I want you to know that Jake is safe right now – he's here with me in my office – but this is something that requires immediate attention and professional help."

Follow-up information to provide:

- Specific statements Jake made (without breaking confidentiality unnecessarily)

- Safety measures you've implemented at school

- Why this requires professional evaluation

- Resources for emergency mental health services

- What will happen if they don't seek immediate help

- Support available to the family during this crisis

Common parent reactions and responses:

"Are you sure? He seemed fine this morning." "I understand this is shocking. Depression and suicidal thoughts often aren't visible to family members because young people work hard to hide their pain. The fact that he seemed fine doesn't mean he wasn't struggling internally."

"What did we do wrong?" "Mental health problems aren't caused by bad parenting. They're complex conditions that can affect any young person, regardless of their family situation. What matters now is getting Jake the help he needs."

"Can't we just watch him more closely at home?" "I appreciate that you want to help Jake yourselves, but suicidal thoughts require

professional evaluation and treatment. This isn't something families should try to handle alone, even with the best intentions."

Self-Harm Discovery Communication

Parents often react with shock, guilt, and fear when they learn their child has been engaging in self-harm behaviors.

Script for self-harm notification: "Mrs. Garcia, I'm calling about Sofia because I discovered today that she's been engaging in some self-harm behaviors – specifically cutting on her arms. I want to assure you first that her injuries aren't life-threatening and I've provided appropriate medical care. But I'm concerned about what this tells us about her emotional state, and I think it's important for us to work together to get her additional support."

Information to provide:

- Medical status of any injuries (treated, healing, not serious)
- What you understand about why she's engaging in self-harm
- Safety planning you've done at school
- Recommendations for mental health evaluation
- Resources for parents dealing with self-harm behaviors
- Follow-up plans and monitoring

Address common parent concerns:

About secrecy: "Many young people keep self-harm behaviors secret because they feel ashamed or worried about how adults will react. This doesn't mean Sofia doesn't trust you – it means she's been struggling and didn't know how to ask for help."

About escalation: "Self-harm behaviors can be serious even when they're not intended to be lethal. They often indicate significant

177

emotional distress and can escalate over time, which is why professional help is important."

About treatment: "There are effective treatments for self-harm behaviors. Many young people learn healthier coping strategies and stop engaging in self-harm with appropriate support."

Recommendation for Evaluation Scripts

When recommending professional mental health evaluation, parents need to understand why this is necessary and what it involves.

Script for evaluation recommendations: "Based on my assessment of Michael's symptoms – the persistent sadness, difficulty sleeping, loss of interest in activities, and trouble concentrating – I'm recommending that you have him evaluated by a mental health professional. This doesn't mean there's anything seriously wrong with him, but these symptoms suggest he might be struggling with depression, and early intervention can make a big difference in how quickly he feels better."

Explain what evaluation involves:

- Meeting with a trained mental health professional
- Assessment of symptoms, functioning, and risk factors
- Discussion of treatment options if needed
- Development of a plan for ongoing support
- Coordination with school staff as appropriate

Address evaluation concerns:

"Will this go on his permanent record?" "Mental health treatment is confidential medical care. It doesn't become part of his school record unless you specifically request accommodations that require school involvement."

"Are you saying he needs medication?" "Evaluation helps determine what types of support would be most helpful. Many young people benefit from counseling without needing medication, while others do well with a combination of therapy and medication. The evaluation helps figure out what's right for Michael specifically."

Managing Resistant Parents

Some parents respond to mental health concerns with denial, minimization, or outright refusal to seek help. Your approach needs to address their resistance while still advocating for the student's needs.

"My Child is Fine" Responses

When parents insist their child doesn't have mental health concerns despite evidence to the contrary, you need strategies that don't create defensiveness while still communicating your concerns.

Responding to denial: "I can understand why this might be hard to believe, especially since children often work really hard to seem okay around their families. Let me share some specific things I've observed at school that concern me, and then I'd love to hear your perspective on how things have been at home."

Provide specific examples: Instead of saying "She seems depressed," say "Over the past three weeks, I've noticed that Sarah comes to my office almost daily with headaches or stomach pain, she's eating very little at lunch, and her teachers report she's not participating in class discussions like she used to."

Ask for parent input: "Have you noticed any changes in her sleep patterns, appetite, or interest in activities she usually enjoys?" This approach invites collaboration rather than confrontation.

Acknowledge their perspective: "It sounds like she's still functioning well at home, which is actually pretty common with depression in teenagers. They often use all their energy to seem normal at home and then struggle more at school."

Stigma and Denial Addressing

Cultural stigma, personal beliefs, and fear can lead parents to deny or minimize mental health concerns.

Addressing stigma directly: "I know that mental health concerns can feel scary or shameful in some families or cultures. But just like we wouldn't ignore signs of diabetes or asthma, we can't ignore signs that suggest emotional distress. Getting help early actually prevents more serious problems later."

Reframe mental health: "Mental health is really just part of overall health. When we take care of physical health with regular checkups and treatment when needed, we're doing the same thing with mental health."

Address specific stigma concerns:

"Mental health problems mean weakness" "Actually, dealing with mental health challenges takes incredible strength. And getting help when you need it shows wisdom and courage, not weakness."

"This will ruin their future" "Getting help for mental health concerns actually protects their future. Young people who receive appropriate support do much better academically and socially than those who struggle without help."

"People will find out and judge us" "Mental health treatment is confidential medical care. The only people who need to know are those directly involved in helping your child."

Legal Obligation Explanations

Sometimes you need to explain to parents what your legal obligations are when they refuse to seek appropriate help for their child.

Explaining mandatory reporting: "I understand you prefer to handle this within the family, and I respect that preference. However,

I have legal obligations to ensure student safety. If I believe a child is at risk and parents aren't seeking appropriate help, I may need to involve other agencies to ensure the child's safety."

Clarifying when reporting is required: "I'm not required to report mental health concerns themselves, but I am required to report situations where a child's safety is at risk and they're not receiving appropriate care. Right now, I'm hoping we can work together to get [child's name] the help they need."

Making legal obligations collaborative: "Let's figure out together how to get [child's name] the support they need. I want to work with you on this, and I'm hoping we can find a solution that feels comfortable for your family while still addressing my concerns about their safety."

Compromise Strategies

When parents are resistant to your initial recommendations, look for compromise solutions that still address the student's needs.

Graduated approach: "I understand you're not ready for formal mental health counseling right now. Would you be open to starting with your family doctor or pediatrician? They can do an initial assessment and help determine next steps."

Time-limited agreements: "What if we try some school-based support for the next month and then reassess? If things don't improve, would you be willing to consider outside counseling at that point?"

Family-friendly alternatives: "I know individual therapy feels intimidating. Some families find family counseling or support groups less overwhelming as a starting point."

Cultural adaptations: "Are there cultural or religious leaders in your community who might be able to provide support while we're also working on the mental health aspects?"

Resource Provision Conversations

Parents need concrete, practical information about how to access mental health services, but they also need guidance about navigating complex systems.

Insurance Navigation Discussions

Many families don't understand how mental health coverage works or what their insurance will pay for.

Basic insurance information to provide: "Most insurance plans are required to cover mental health treatment at the same level as physical health treatment. Let me give you some questions to ask when you call your insurance company."

Questions for parents to ask insurance:

- "What is my copay for mental health visits?"
- "Do I need a referral from my primary care doctor?"
- "Which mental health providers in our area accept our insurance?"
- "How many therapy sessions are covered per year?"
- "Is there a separate deductible for mental health services?"
- "What's the difference between in-network and out-of-network coverage?"

For families without insurance:

- Community mental health centers that offer sliding-scale fees
- University training clinics that provide lower-cost services
- Crisis services that are available regardless of insurance status
- State and local programs for children's mental health services
- Online therapy options that may be more affordable

Community Resource Introductions

Parents need to understand what different types of mental health services are available and how to choose appropriate care.

Types of mental health services to explain:

- Individual therapy (one-on-one counseling)
- Family therapy (involving multiple family members)
- Group therapy (with other young people facing similar challenges)
- Intensive outpatient programs (multiple sessions per week)
- Psychiatric medication evaluation and management
- Crisis intervention services

How to choose a provider: "Look for someone who specializes in working with teenagers and has experience with the specific concerns we've discussed. You can ask potential therapists about their training and approach during initial phone calls."

Questions parents can ask potential providers:

- "What experience do you have working with teenagers?"
- "What's your approach to treating [specific condition]?"
- "How do you involve families in treatment?"
- "What should we expect from therapy sessions?"
- "How will we know if treatment is working?"

School-Based Service Explanations

Parents need to understand what mental health support is available at school and how it coordinates with outside treatment.

School-based mental health services to explain:

- Individual counseling with school counselors or social workers

- Group counseling or support groups
- Crisis intervention and safety planning
- Academic accommodations for mental health concerns
- Coordination with outside mental health providers
- Peer support programs or mentoring

Benefits of school-based services:

- Easily accessible during school hours
- No cost to families
- Integrated with academic support
- Familiar environment for students
- Coordination with teachers and other school staff

Limitations of school-based services:

- Limited time available for individual students
- Focus on school-related functioning rather than comprehensive treatment
- May not be sufficient for serious mental health concerns
- Staff may not have specialized training in specific conditions

How school and outside services work together: "School-based support and outside therapy work best when they're coordinated. With your permission, I can communicate with outside providers to ensure everyone is working toward the same goals for your child."

Chapter 4.3: Staff Communication

Your phone rings at 11:30 AM. It's Jake's math teacher, and she sounds frustrated. "Jake has been in my class for three months, and something is seriously wrong with him. He sleeps through half my lessons, never turns in homework, and yesterday he got angry and stormed out when I asked him a simple question. I don't know if this is a discipline problem, a learning problem, or what, but I need help."

You know that Jake has been struggling with depression and anxiety, that his parents are going through a difficult divorce, and that he's been working with the school counselor on coping strategies. But you also know that his teacher needs specific, practical information about how to support him without violating his privacy or making him feel singled out.

Staff communication about student mental health requires you to balance multiple competing needs: the student's right to privacy, the teacher's need for information to provide appropriate support, administrators' need to understand resource allocation and safety concerns, and the broader team's need for coordination. You're often the hub that connects all these different perspectives and needs.

Teacher Notification Templates

Teachers spend more time with students than any other school staff, which makes them crucial partners in supporting student mental health. But they're also busy, often overwhelmed, and may not have training in mental health issues. Your communication needs to be clear, practical, and respectful of their expertise in education.

What Teachers Need to Know

Teachers don't need diagnostic information or detailed personal history, but they do need practical information that helps them understand and support the student in their classroom.

Essential information for teachers:

- Brief, general description of what the student is dealing with ("managing some anxiety" or "working through some depression")

- How mental health concerns might show up in the classroom (difficulty concentrating, increased absences, emotional outbursts, social withdrawal)

- Specific accommodations or modifications that would be helpful

- Warning signs that indicate the student needs additional support

- Who to contact if concerns arise and how urgently to respond

Information teachers typically don't need:

- Specific diagnosis or detailed symptom lists

- Family dynamics or personal history

- Details about therapy or medication

- Information about other students involved in the situation

- Specific incidents that led to mental health concerns

Sample teacher notification: "I wanted to let you know that Maria has been working with me and the counselor on managing some anxiety that's been affecting her school performance. You might notice that she sometimes seems worried or overwhelmed, especially during tests or presentations. She's learning some coping strategies, but it would be helpful if you could check in with her briefly after class on days when she seems particularly stressed. If you notice signs that she's really struggling – like refusing to participate, seeming panicked, or asking to leave class frequently – please send her to me so I can help her use her coping strategies."

Confidentiality Boundaries

Teachers have legitimate educational interests in information that affects classroom performance and safety, but you need to be clear about what information can and cannot be shared.

Information you can share without specific consent:

- General categories of mental health concerns that affect educational performance
- Specific accommodations that are needed in the classroom
- Behavioral strategies that are helpful for the student
- Warning signs to watch for that indicate need for additional support
- Emergency procedures if the student is in crisis

Information that requires specific consent:

- Detailed diagnostic information
- Specific therapy goals or treatment plans
- Family dynamics or personal history
- Information about other family members' mental health
- Specific medication information beyond basic side effects

How to maintain confidentiality while providing useful information: "I can't share specific details about Sam's situation, but I can tell you that he's dealing with some mental health concerns that sometimes make it hard for him to concentrate and stay organized.

He's working on strategies to manage this, and here's how you can support him in your classroom..."

Accommodation Recommendations

Teachers need specific, actionable suggestions for how to modify their classroom approach to support students with mental health concerns.

Academic accommodations:

- Extended time on tests and assignments
- Alternative testing locations (quiet, private spaces)
- Reduced homework load or modified assignments
- Flexibility with due dates during mental health episodes
- Permission to take breaks during class
- Alternative participation formats (written vs. oral responses)

Environmental accommodations:

- Seating preferences (near door, away from distractions, with supportive peers)
- Reduced stimulation during overwhelming periods
- Access to calming tools (fidget items, stress balls)
- Permission to use coping strategies during class (breathing exercises, brief walks)
- Modified expectations during crisis periods

Social accommodations:

- Flexibility with group work requirements
- Support for peer relationship difficulties
- Modified participation in social activities

- Protection from bullying or stigma related to mental health

- Assistance with communication skills

Sample accommodation communication: "David is working on managing depression that sometimes makes it difficult for him to concentrate and complete tasks. During his more difficult periods, it would be helpful if you could: allow him extra time on assignments, check in with him privately about his understanding of material rather than calling on him in class, and let him know he can take a brief walk in the hallway if he's feeling overwhelmed. If you notice that he's not participating at all or seems particularly withdrawn for several days in a row, please let me know."

Behavioral Observation Requests

Sometimes you need teachers to watch for specific behaviors or changes that might indicate worsening mental health or improvement with interventions.

What to ask teachers to observe:

- Changes in academic performance or participation

- Social interactions and peer relationships

- Emotional regulation and coping strategies

- Physical symptoms that might be related to mental health

- Response to accommodations and interventions

How to make observation requests: "As we work with Emma on her anxiety management, it would be helpful if you could keep an eye on how she's doing with class presentations and group work. I'm particularly interested in whether the breathing techniques we've taught her seem to be helping, and whether her anxiety seems to be getting better, worse, or staying about the same. You don't need to do anything formal – just let me know if you notice significant changes in either direction."

Making observations manageable for busy teachers:

- Focus on specific, observable behaviors rather than internal states

- Provide simple rating scales or checklists when appropriate

- Ask for observations over time periods (weekly updates) rather than daily reports

- Connect observations to things teachers are already noticing in their classroom management

Administrator Briefing Protocols

Administrators need different information than teachers because they're responsible for policy decisions, resource allocation, safety oversight, and legal compliance.

Crisis Situation Updates

When students are experiencing mental health crises, administrators need timely, accurate information that helps them make appropriate decisions about safety, resources, and communication.

Information administrators need during crises:

- Nature and severity of the crisis (suicide risk, aggressive behavior, psychotic episode)

- Immediate safety measures that have been implemented

- Students and staff who are directly affected

- Parents who have been contacted and their responses

- Outside agencies or professionals who have been involved

- Resources or support that may be needed

- Anticipated timeline for resolution

Sample crisis update: "I'm updating you on the situation with Alex Thompson, the 10th grader who was referred for suicide risk this morning. I completed a risk assessment and determined he has moderate risk with some planning but no immediate intent. I've implemented 1:1 supervision and contacted his parents, who are cooperating and taking him for emergency evaluation this afternoon. His English and math teachers have been briefly informed that he won't be in their classes today but will return tomorrow with additional support. No other students were directly involved. I'll follow up tomorrow morning about his status and any accommodations he might need."

Resource Need Communications

Administrators make decisions about staffing, funding, and program development based partly on information about student mental health needs and resource gaps.

Resource needs to communicate:

- Patterns in mental health referrals and crises

- Gaps in available services or support

- Staff training needs related to mental health

- Space or equipment needs for mental health services

- Coordination challenges with outside providers

- Success stories and positive outcomes from current programs

Sample resource need communication: "Over the past month, I've seen a 40% increase in students requesting mental health support, particularly related to anxiety and depression. Our current counseling resources are stretched thin, and I'm having to refer more students to outside providers, which creates delays in getting help. I think we should consider whether additional mental health staffing or expanded partnerships with community providers might help us meet this increased need."

Policy Issue Identification

When you identify school policies that create barriers to effective mental health support, administrators need to understand the issue and potential solutions.

Policy issues that might need administrative attention:

- Disciplinary policies that don't account for mental health factors

- Attendance policies that penalize students for mental health-related absences

- Academic policies that don't provide adequate accommodations

- Communication policies that create barriers to coordinating care

- Safety protocols that may not address mental health crises effectively

How to present policy concerns: "I've been working with several students whose depression causes them to miss significant amounts of school. Our current attendance policy doesn't distinguish between unexcused absences and absences related to mental health treatment, which means these students are facing truancy consequences even when they're actively working on their mental health. I'd like to discuss how we might modify our approach to better support students who are receiving mental health treatment."

Multidisciplinary Team Communication

Students with mental health concerns often need support from multiple school professionals, outside providers, and family members. Coordinating this team requires clear communication protocols and shared understanding of roles.

Case Presentation Formats

When presenting student cases to multidisciplinary teams, you need to organize information in ways that facilitate decision-making and coordination.

Standard case presentation format:

1. **Student identification:** Name, grade, relevant demographic information

2. **Presenting concerns:** Current symptoms, behaviors, or crises that prompted referral

3. **Background:** Relevant history, family situation, previous interventions

4. **Assessment results:** Screening tools, observations, risk assessments

5. **Current interventions:** What's being done now and how it's working

6. **Recommendations:** What additional support or changes are needed

7. **Team member roles:** Who will do what and when

Sample case presentation opening: "I'm presenting the case of Jordan Martinez, a 14-year-old 9th grader who was referred last week for increasing anxiety and school avoidance. Over the past month, Jordan has missed 12 days of school, visited my office daily with physical complaints like headaches and stomach pain, and has been refusing to attend his math and science classes. His parents report that he's been having trouble sleeping and has expressed fears about 'failing everything' and 'disappointing everyone.'"

Progress Reporting Templates

Regular team meetings need structured progress updates that help track student improvement and adjust interventions as needed.

Progress report elements:

- Student response to current interventions
- New concerns or changes in presentation
- Family engagement and feedback
- Academic and social functioning updates
- Coordination with outside providers
- Modifications needed to current plan
- Goals for upcoming time period

Sample progress report: "Update on Sarah Chen: Over the past two weeks, Sarah has used her coping strategies successfully in 3 out of 4 instances when she felt panicked during class. She's attended all her classes and completed most assignments with the extended time accommodation. Her parents report improved sleep and less morning anxiety. Her therapist notes good engagement in sessions. Goals for next two weeks: continue current accommodations, begin gradual exposure to presentation activities, and maintain weekly check-ins with counselor."

Concern Escalation Protocols

Team members need clear procedures for communicating when student situations become more serious or when current interventions aren't working.

When to escalate concerns:

- Student safety risk has increased
- Current interventions aren't showing expected progress after reasonable time
- New symptoms or behaviors have emerged
- Family situation has changed significantly
- Outside provider has recommended different level of care

- Student is requesting changes to their support plan

How to escalate effectively:

- Provide specific information about what has changed

- Explain why current interventions may not be sufficient

- Suggest specific alternatives or modifications

- Indicate urgency level and timeline for response

- Identify who else needs to be involved in decision-making

Sample concern escalation: "I need to escalate concerns about Michael Rodriguez. Despite implementing our behavior plan three weeks ago, his aggressive outbursts have increased from 2-3 per week to daily episodes. Yesterday's incident involved throwing furniture and required administrator intervention. His parents are requesting a meeting to discuss alternative placement options. I recommend we convene an emergency team meeting to reassess his needs and consider more intensive interventions. This should happen within the next 48 hours given the safety concerns."

Mastering the Art of Therapeutic Communication

Throughout this section, you've gained specific scripts and strategies for the most challenging conversations you'll face as a school nurse addressing mental health concerns. But beyond the specific words and techniques, the underlying skill you're developing is therapeutic communication – the ability to create healing relationships through your interactions with students, families, and colleagues.

Therapeutic communication isn't just about having the right words (though that helps). It's about bringing authenticity, curiosity, and genuine care to every interaction while maintaining appropriate professional boundaries. It's about understanding that how you say something matters as much as what you say, and that sometimes the

195

most therapeutic thing you can do is simply listen with complete presence and attention.

Your communication skills will continue to develop throughout your career as you encounter different students, families, and situations that challenge you to grow. The scripts and strategies in this section provide a foundation, but the real learning happens in the moments when you're sitting across from a struggling teenager or talking with worried parents, using your clinical judgment to adapt your approach to their unique needs and circumstances.

Most importantly, your communication creates the foundation for all the other mental health support you provide. Students won't benefit from your crisis intervention skills if they don't trust you enough to share their struggles. Parents won't follow through on mental health recommendations if they don't feel heard and understood. Teachers won't implement accommodations effectively if they don't have clear, practical information about how to help.

The investment you make in developing excellent communication skills pays dividends in every aspect of your school nursing practice. You're not just sharing information – you're creating relationships that have the power to change lives.

Section 5: Resource Mapping Your Community

Chapter 5.1: Building Your Resource Database

You're sitting in your office at 3:45 PM when Mrs. Chen calls, her voice tight with worry. "The psychiatrist says my daughter needs intensive outpatient therapy for her eating disorder, but I don't even know where to start looking. Do you know anyone who works with teenagers? Someone who takes our insurance? Someone who actually has openings?" You want to help immediately, but you find yourself scrambling through scattered business cards, outdated phone numbers, and half-remembered recommendations from colleagues.

This scenario plays out in school nursing offices across the country every single day. A student needs specialized mental health services, parents are desperate for guidance, and school nurses find themselves trying to provide resource information from incomplete, outdated, or poorly organized systems. You might know there's a good therapist "somewhere across town" or remember hearing about a support group "that meets on weekends," but when families need concrete, actionable information right now, vague recollections aren't enough.

Building a systematic resource database isn't just about organization – it's about ensuring that the students you identify as needing help can actually access that help quickly and effectively. Research shows that the longer the delay between identifying mental health needs and connecting with appropriate services, the less likely families are to follow through. When you can immediately provide specific names, phone numbers, insurance information, and realistic timelines, you transform from someone who "knows about resources" to someone who actually connects students with life-changing support.

12-Week Implementation Plan

Creating a useful resource database requires systematic effort over time. Trying to build it all at once leads to incomplete information, missed connections, and a system that becomes outdated before you finish creating it. A 12-week plan gives you time to be thorough while creating momentum that carries you through to completion.

Week 1-2: Team Formation and Planning

You can't build a resource database alone, nor should you try. The most effective resource systems are created by teams that bring different perspectives and connections to the process.

Identify your core team members:

- School counselors and social workers (they know what types of referrals are most common)

- Special education staff (they understand specialized services and accommodations)

- Administration representative (they can support your efforts and address policy issues)

- Parent coordinator or family liaison (they understand barriers families face)

- Community health nurse or public health representative if available

Essential planning activities:

- Define the scope of your database (age ranges, types of services, geographic boundaries)

- Establish roles and responsibilities for each team member

- Set realistic timelines and meeting schedules

- Identify existing resources that team members already know about

- Determine your target format (digital database, printed guides, or both)

- Establish quality standards for information gathering

Create your foundational framework: Before you start gathering information, decide what information you'll collect about each resource and how you'll organize it. This framework needs to be comprehensive enough to be useful but not so complex that it becomes unwieldy.

Basic information categories:

- Organization/provider name and contact information
- Services provided and populations served
- Insurance accepted and payment options
- Location and transportation considerations
- Wait times and availability
- Application or referral processes
- Cultural and linguistic capabilities

Week 3-6: Resource Inventory Development

These four weeks are your intensive information-gathering phase. Each team member should focus on different categories of resources to avoid duplication while ensuring comprehensive coverage.

Information gathering assignments by team member:

- *School nurse:* Medical providers, crisis services, specialized medical mental health programs
- *Counselor:* Individual and family therapy providers, support groups, educational advocates
- *Social worker:* Community mental health centers, social services, housing and basic needs resources
- *Special education staff:* Disability-specific services, developmental and learning support programs

- *Parent representative:* Parent support groups, family resources, transportation and childcare support

Start with existing connections: Every team member already knows some resources through their professional experience. Begin by documenting these known resources thoroughly, then use them as starting points to discover additional services.

Use systematic discovery methods:

- Contact your local community mental health center for comprehensive provider lists

- Review your county's mental health and social services directory

- Connect with local hospitals and ask for their mental health resource lists

- Contact insurance companies operating in your area for provider directories

- Research nonprofit organizations focused on mental health, family support, and child welfare

- Review online directories like Psychology Today, but verify all information independently

Week 7-10: Verification and Relationship Building

Raw information isn't useful until it's verified and enhanced through direct contact with providers. These weeks focus on turning basic contact information into actionable, accurate resource descriptions.

Verification activities for each resource:

- Call to confirm contact information, services, and availability

- Ask about current wait times and intake processes

- Verify insurance acceptance and payment options

- Inquire about cultural competency and language capabilities

- Understand their referral preferences and requirements

- Ask about their experience working with school-age children

Build relationships during verification: Don't just collect information – introduce yourself and your role. Explain that you're building a resource database to better serve students and families. Many providers appreciate knowing about school nurses who are actively connecting students with services.

Key relationship-building activities:

- Introduce yourself and your school during every contact

- Explain your role in student mental health and your referral volume

- Ask providers what information would be helpful for them to receive with referrals

- Invite providers to visit your school or meet with your mental health team

- Ask about their availability for consultation on difficult cases

- Exchange business cards and establish preferred communication methods

Week 11-12: Database Creation and Training

The final two weeks focus on organizing your collected information into usable formats and training team members to use and maintain the system.

Database organization priorities:

- Create user-friendly formats that can be quickly accessed during crisis situations

- Develop multiple organization systems (by service type, by insurance, by location)
- Build in regular update and maintenance schedules
- Ensure information is accessible to everyone who needs it
- Create backup systems and redundancy for critical resources

Training components for all team members:

- How to access and search the database efficiently
- Protocols for updating information and adding new resources
- Standards for sharing resource information with families
- Procedures for tracking referral outcomes and provider feedback
- Systems for identifying gaps in services and finding new resources

Essential Resource Categories

A useful mental health resource database needs to be comprehensive enough to address the full range of needs you'll encounter, from immediate crisis intervention to long-term therapeutic support.

Crisis Services

Crisis services are your safety net – the resources you turn to when students are in immediate danger or when situations can't wait for regular appointment scheduling.

Crisis hotlines: National crisis hotlines provide 24/7 support for students experiencing suicidal thoughts, severe depression, or overwhelming anxiety. Document not just phone numbers, but also text and chat options that many teenagers prefer.

Essential crisis hotlines to include:

- 988 Suicide & Crisis Lifeline (nationwide, 24/7)

- Crisis Text Line (text HOME to 741741)

- Local crisis hotlines specific to your community

- Specialized hotlines (LGBTQ+ specific, eating disorders, substance abuse)

- Teen-specific crisis lines that use peer counselors

Information to collect for each hotline:

- Phone number, text options, and website

- Languages supported beyond English

- Specific training of staff (teen-focused, trauma-informed, culturally competent)

- Whether they provide follow-up support or just crisis intervention

- How they coordinate with local emergency services

Mobile crisis teams: Many communities now have mobile crisis teams that can respond to schools or homes when students are in psychiatric crisis. These teams can often provide immediate assessment and intervention without requiring emergency room visits.

Information to document:

- Service area and response times

- Age ranges served (some teams only serve adults)

- How to request services and who can make requests

- What types of situations they respond to

- Whether they can transport students for evaluation

- Cost and insurance coverage

Outpatient Mental Health Providers

Outpatient therapy is the foundation of most mental health treatment for students. Your database needs to provide families with realistic options that match their needs, insurance, and preferences.

Individual therapy providers: Document therapists who specialize in child and adolescent mental health, with particular attention to those who have experience with school-age concerns like academic anxiety, peer relationships, and family dynamics.

Critical information for therapy providers:

- Specializations and treatment approaches (CBT, family therapy, trauma-focused)

- Age ranges served (many adult therapists don't work with teenagers)

- Insurance accepted and sliding scale options

- Current wait times for new patients

- Location and transportation accessibility

- Cultural competency and languages spoken

Psychiatric medication management: Many students benefit from psychiatric medications in combination with therapy. Document providers who can prescribe and monitor psychiatric medications for children and adolescents.

Medication management information:

- Child/adolescent psychiatrists vs. general psychiatrists willing to see teens

- Nurse practitioners with psychiatric prescribing authority

- Primary care providers who prescribe psychiatric medications

- Medication clinics and their specializations

- Coordination requirements with therapy providers

Specialized Programs

Some mental health conditions require specialized treatment approaches that aren't available through general therapy providers. Your database needs to identify these specialized resources and their specific admission requirements.

Eating disorder treatment: Eating disorders require specialized treatment that addresses both the psychological and medical aspects of these conditions. Document providers who have specific training and experience in eating disorder treatment.

Eating disorder resource information:

- Outpatient eating disorder therapists
- Registered dietitians who work with eating disorders
- Medical providers who monitor eating disorder patients
- Intensive outpatient programs (IOP) for eating disorders
- Residential treatment programs and their admission criteria
- Support groups for eating disorders and family members

Substance abuse treatment: Adolescent substance abuse treatment requires specialized approaches that differ significantly from adult treatment programs. Document both traditional treatment programs and newer approaches that recognize substance use as often co-occurring with mental health issues.

Substance abuse resources:

- Adolescent-specific outpatient treatment programs
- Inpatient/residential substance abuse programs for teens
- Dual diagnosis programs that address both mental health and substance use
- Medication-assisted treatment options for adolescents

- Family programs that support parents of teens with substance abuse issues

- Peer recovery support programs for teenagers

Support Services

Mental health treatment is most effective when it's supported by additional services that address the broader needs of students and families.

Peer support programs: Many teenagers benefit from connecting with other young people who have faced similar mental health challenges. Document peer support programs that provide safe, structured environments for these connections.

Family therapy and support: Mental health challenges affect entire families, and many students benefit when family members are involved in treatment. Document resources that specifically work with families around mental health issues.

Family support resources:

- Family therapy providers who specialize in adolescent mental health

- Support groups for parents of teenagers with mental health challenges

- Educational workshops about adolescent mental health for families

- Respite care services for families dealing with intensive mental health needs

- Sibling support groups and resources

Social Services

Mental health problems are often complicated by social and economic factors. Your database needs to include resources that address these underlying issues that can interfere with mental health treatment.

Housing and basic needs: Students experiencing homelessness or housing instability have significantly higher rates of mental health problems. Document resources that can provide stable housing and basic needs support.

Educational support: Some students need educational advocacy or specialized educational services as part of their mental health treatment. Document resources that understand the intersection between mental health and educational needs.

Information Gathering Templates

Systematic information collection requires standardized templates that ensure you gather the same essential information about every resource. These templates also help you update information efficiently when resources change.

Provider Information Sheets

Create standardized forms that capture all essential information about each mental health provider or service. Consistency in information gathering makes your database more useful and easier to maintain.

Basic provider information template:

Contact Information:

- Organization/provider name
- Primary contact person and title
- Phone number(s) and best times to call
- Email address and website
- Physical address and directions
- Mailing address if different

Services and Specializations:

- Primary services offered

- Age ranges served

- Specific mental health specializations

- Treatment approaches used

- Languages spoken by providers

- Cultural competencies

Practical Information:

- Insurance plans accepted

- Self-pay rates and sliding scale options

- Current wait times for new patients

- Intake process and requirements

- Referral requirements (doctor referral needed?)

- Transportation accessibility

Service Verification Checklists

Use verification checklists to ensure you've confirmed essential information and haven't missed critical details during your provider contacts.

Verification checklist items:

- Confirmed contact information is current

- Verified services offered match what's advertised

- Confirmed age ranges and populations served

- Checked current availability and wait times

- Verified insurance acceptance and payment options

- Confirmed location and accessibility

- Asked about referral preferences and requirements

- Inquired about consultation availability for complex cases

Insurance and Payment Grids

Create charts that help families quickly identify which providers accept their insurance or offer affordable payment options.

Payment information to track:

- Major insurance plans accepted (list specific plans, not just "most insurance")

- Medicaid acceptance and any restrictions

- Self-pay rates for different services

- Sliding scale availability and qualification requirements

- Payment plan options

- Copay amounts for different insurance plans

- Coverage for different types of services (individual therapy, family therapy, psychiatric evaluation)

Wait Time Tracking Systems

Wait times for mental health services can change rapidly, especially for specialized providers. Build systems to track and update wait time information regularly.

Wait time categories:

- Crisis/urgent appointments (same day or within 1-2 days)

- Standard new patient appointments

- Specialized services (eating disorders, trauma therapy)

- Medication management appointments

- Family therapy or group therapy
- Seasonal variations in wait times

Update wait time information:

- Monthly for high-volume providers
- Quarterly for specialized services
- After major changes in community mental health resources
- At the beginning of each school year when demand typically increases

Chapter 5.2: Relationship Building Strategies

Having accurate information about mental health resources is only the first step. The real effectiveness of your resource database depends on the relationships you build with providers and the ongoing partnerships you maintain. A provider who knows you, understands your student population, and trusts your clinical judgment will be much more responsive to your referrals than one who only knows you as a name on a referral form.

Think of resource building as networking with a purpose. You're not just collecting business cards – you're creating professional relationships that will directly benefit the students and families you serve. When a provider knows that referrals from your school are well-screened and appropriately matched, they're more likely to prioritize your students, provide consultation when you have questions, and work collaboratively to ensure successful treatment outcomes.

Provider Outreach Protocols

Reaching out to mental health providers requires a professional approach that clearly communicates your role, your student population's needs, and how partnership with your school can be mutually beneficial.

Introduction Letter Templates

Your initial contact with providers sets the tone for your ongoing relationship. A well-crafted introduction letter positions you as a professional colleague rather than just another referral source.

Sample introduction letter framework:

Dear [Provider Name],

My name is [Your Name], and I'm the school nurse at [School Name], serving [number] students in grades [range]. I'm reaching out because I understand that you provide [specific services] and I'm building a resource database to better connect our students and families with appropriate mental health support.

In my role, I regularly work with students experiencing [mention common issues you see – anxiety, depression, trauma, family stress]. I conduct mental health screenings, provide crisis intervention, and coordinate care with outside providers to ensure students receive comprehensive support.

I'd appreciate the opportunity to learn more about your services and discuss how we might work together to support students in our community. Specifically, I'm hoping to understand:

- *Your specializations and treatment approaches*
- *Current availability for new patients*
- *Insurance and payment options*
- *Your preferences for receiving referral information*
- *Whether you're available for consultation on complex cases*

I'm happy to schedule a brief meeting at your convenience, or we can start with a phone conversation. I believe that strong partnerships between schools and community mental health providers lead to better outcomes for the young people we all serve.

Thank you for your time and for the important work you do with children and adolescents in our community.

Sincerely, [Your name and credentials] [Contact information]

Meeting Agenda Suggestions

When providers agree to meet with you, come prepared with a structured agenda that respects their time while gathering the information you need.

Standard meeting agenda:

1. **Introduction and context** (5 minutes)
   - Your role and student population
   - Current mental health needs you're seeing
   - Your approach to connecting families with resources

2. **Provider services and approach** (10 minutes)
   - Services offered and specializations
   - Treatment philosophy and approaches
   - Experience with school-age populations
   - Cultural competency and language capabilities

3. **Practical information** (10 minutes)
   - Current availability and wait times
   - Insurance acceptance and payment options
   - Intake process and referral requirements
   - Location and accessibility considerations

4. **Collaboration opportunities** (10 minutes)
   - Preferences for receiving referral information
   - Availability for consultation on complex cases
   - Interest in school-based presentations or training
   - Communication preferences and protocols

5. **Next steps and follow-up** (5 minutes)
   - How you'll include them in your resource database
   - Plans for ongoing communication

   o Timeline for potential first referrals

Collaboration Agreement Templates

Formal collaboration agreements help clarify expectations and establish professional protocols for working together effectively.

Elements of effective collaboration agreements:

- Scope of services the provider offers to your students
- Referral processes and required information
- Communication protocols for ongoing cases
- Emergency consultation availability
- Information sharing agreements (with appropriate consent)
- Quality assurance and feedback mechanisms
- Review and renewal timelines for the agreement

Sample collaboration agreement outline:

This agreement establishes a collaborative relationship between [School Name] and [Provider Name] to support the mental health needs of students and families in our community.

Referral Process:

- School will provide detailed referral information including assessment results, school observations, and family contact information
- Provider will acknowledge receipt of referrals within [timeframe]
- Provider will provide general updates on student progress (with appropriate consent)

Communication Protocols:

- School designates [specific person] as primary contact for this provider

- Provider designates [specific person] as primary school contact

- Emergency consultation available during [specified hours] at [contact method]

- Regular communication about service availability and any changes to programs

Professional Standards:

- Both parties maintain appropriate confidentiality and informed consent procedures

- All communications comply with FERPA and HIPAA requirements

- Services provided according to relevant professional and ethical standards

Maintaining Partnerships

Building relationships is only the beginning – maintaining effective partnerships requires ongoing effort and systematic attention to the health of your provider network.

Regular Check-in Schedules

Consistent communication keeps your relationships strong and your information current. Different types of providers need different communication schedules based on how frequently you work together.

Monthly check-ins for high-volume providers:

- Providers you refer to frequently (more than 2-3 students per month)

- Crisis services that you need to access quickly

- Primary mental health partners for your school

Monthly check-in agenda:

- Current wait times and availability
- Any changes to services or policies
- Feedback on recent referrals
- Updates on community mental health needs
- Upcoming training or collaboration opportunities

Quarterly check-ins for moderate-use providers:

- Specialized services you use occasionally
- Providers with specific expertise you need periodically
- Backup resources for when primary providers are unavailable

Quarterly check-in agenda:

- Confirm contact information and services
- Update wait times and availability
- Review any changes in insurance acceptance or payment policies
- Discuss any concerns or suggestions for improving referral process

Annual reviews for all providers:

- Complete review of all information in your database
- Assessment of partnership effectiveness
- Planning for the upcoming year's mental health needs
- Formal evaluation of collaboration agreements

Referral Feedback Systems

Systematic feedback helps you improve your referral process and strengthens relationships with providers who feel heard and valued.

Feedback to gather from providers:

- Quality and usefulness of referral information you provide
- Appropriateness of referral matches
- Communication effectiveness
- Suggestions for improving collaboration
- Changes in their services or availability

Feedback to request about outcomes:

- General progress of students you've referred (with appropriate consent)
- Successful interventions or strategies that worked well
- Challenges or barriers that interfered with treatment
- Recommendations for supporting students during treatment
- Suggestions for prevention or early intervention strategies

Feedback systems to implement:

- Brief email surveys after major referrals
- Annual feedback meetings with key providers
- Informal check-ins during regular communication
- Participation in community mental health feedback systems

Joint Training Opportunities

Shared learning experiences strengthen partnerships while improving the quality of care students receive from both school and community providers.

Training topics that benefit both schools and providers:

218

- Adolescent development and mental health

- Cultural competency in mental health services

- Trauma-informed approaches to student support

- Crisis intervention and suicide prevention

- Family engagement strategies

- Coordination between school and clinical services

Types of joint training to organize:

- Provider presentations to school staff about their services

- School presentations to providers about educational environment and student needs

- Shared participation in community mental health conferences

- Case consultation meetings that provide learning for everyone involved

- Online webinar series that both schools and providers can access

Appreciation Strategies

Recognizing and appreciating your provider partners helps maintain positive relationships and encourages continued collaboration.

Formal appreciation strategies:

- Annual recognition events for community mental health partners

- Inclusion in school newsletters or communications highlighting community partnerships

- Letters of appreciation to provider supervisors or organizations

- Nominations for community service awards or professional recognition
- Public recognition during school board meetings or community events

Informal appreciation strategies:

- Personal thank-you notes for exceptional service
- Small gifts during holidays or Mental Health Awareness Month
- Sharing success stories (with appropriate consent) that highlight provider contributions
- Referrals to other schools or organizations that might benefit from their services
- Professional references or recommendations when appropriate

Community Coalition Participation

Mental health support for students requires community-wide coordination. Participating in local coalitions and advocacy groups helps you stay informed about resource changes while contributing to systemic improvements in mental health services.

Finding Relevant Coalitions

Most communities have formal or informal groups focused on mental health, child welfare, or family support. Finding and joining relevant coalitions connects you with broader networks of resources and expertise.

Types of coalitions to look for:

- Community mental health coalitions or alliances
- Child and family advocacy groups

- Suicide prevention coalitions

- Substance abuse prevention partnerships

- Educational support networks

- Healthcare coordination groups

How to identify active coalitions:

- Contact your local community mental health center for information about existing groups

- Check with your county health department about public health coalitions

- Ask other school nurses about groups they participate in

- Look for nonprofit organizations that convene community partnerships

- Search local government websites for citizen advisory committees

Coalition participation benefits:

- Access to information about new services and resources

- Opportunities to influence mental health policy and funding

- Professional development and training opportunities

- Networking with other professionals serving similar populations

- Advocacy training and support for systemic change efforts

Representing School Needs

When you participate in community coalitions, you bring a unique perspective about student mental health needs and school-based interventions. Your voice helps ensure that community planning considers school-based perspectives.

School perspectives to contribute:

- Trends in student mental health needs and utilization
- Barriers families face in accessing mental health services
- Effectiveness of different community resources from a school perspective
- Gaps in services for school-age populations
- Successful models of school-community partnership

Information to gather from coalition participation:

- Funding opportunities for school-based mental health programs
- Policy changes that might affect student mental health services
- New resources or programs being developed in your community
- Research and best practices being implemented elsewhere
- Training opportunities for school staff

Advocacy Strategies

Participating in mental health advocacy helps improve the overall system of care for students while building your knowledge of policy and funding issues that affect resource availability.

School-based advocacy priorities:

- Adequate funding for school mental health services
- Training requirements for school staff working with student mental health
- Policies that support coordination between schools and community mental health providers

- Insurance coverage for mental health services for children and adolescents

- Crisis intervention services available to schools

Advocacy activities to consider:

- Writing letters or emails to elected officials about mental health funding and policy

- Participating in advocacy days at state capitals

- Sharing student success stories (with appropriate consent) to demonstrate the importance of mental health services

- Joining professional organizations that engage in policy advocacy

- Speaking at community meetings about student mental health needs

Chapter 5.3: Creating Accessible Resource Guides

Having a comprehensive resource database is only valuable if the information is accessible to the people who need it most – students, families, and school staff. Creating user-friendly resource guides requires thinking carefully about your different audiences, their varying needs, and the most effective ways to present information for each group.

A parent calling you at 4 PM about their teenager's depression crisis needs different information than a teacher trying to find ongoing support resources for a student with anxiety. A 16-year-old researching help for themselves needs a different approach than a 10-year-old's parents looking for family therapy. Your resource guides need to be tailored to these different users while maintaining consistency and accuracy across all formats.

Format Options

Different situations call for different formats of resource information. Build multiple ways for people to access your resource database so they can get the information they need in the format that works best for their situation.

Digital Databases

Online databases provide the most comprehensive and up-to-date resource information, but they need to be designed with user experience in mind to be truly helpful.

Digital database advantages:

- Can include extensive information about each resource
- Easily updated when information changes

- Searchable by multiple criteria (location, insurance, specialization)
- Accessible 24/7 from any internet connection
- Can include links to provider websites and online scheduling
- Cost-effective to maintain and distribute

Digital database design considerations:

- Simple, intuitive search functions that don't require technical expertise
- Mobile-friendly design that works on smartphones and tablets
- Multiple organization options (alphabetical, by service type, by location)
- Clear categories that make sense to users, not just professionals
- Contact information prominently displayed for each resource
- Regular update timestamps so users know information is current

Essential features for digital databases:

- Search filters for insurance, location, age served, and service type
- Brief descriptions that explain what each provider actually does
- Practical information like wait times, transportation options, and languages spoken
- Emergency resources clearly marked and easily accessible
- Print-friendly options for users who prefer physical copies

Printed Quick-Reference Guides

Physical resource guides serve important functions that digital resources can't fully replace, particularly for crisis situations and for families with limited internet access.

When printed guides are most useful:

- Crisis situations where quick access to key resources is essential

- Families without reliable internet access or limited technology skills

- Situations where families want to review options without using devices

- Backup resources when digital systems are unavailable

- Distribution at community events, health fairs, and parent meetings

Printed guide design principles:

- Clear, large fonts that are easy to read under stress

- Logical organization that helps users find information quickly

- Essential information only – too much detail makes guides overwhelming

- Contact information prominently displayed

- Durable materials that can withstand frequent use

- Regular update schedules with clear version dates

Content for printed quick-reference guides:

- Crisis resources (hotlines, emergency services, mobile crisis teams)

- Most commonly needed services (general therapy, psychiatric medication, crisis support)

- Basic information about insurance and payment options

- Transportation and accessibility information

- Clear instructions for getting help immediately

Mobile-Friendly Directories

Many families, especially those with teenagers, prefer accessing information on their smartphones. Mobile-optimized resources need to be designed specifically for small screens and touch navigation.

Mobile optimization requirements:

- Fast loading times even with limited data connections

- Large, easily tappable buttons and links

- Simplified navigation that works with thumbs, not mouse clicks

- Click-to-call functionality for phone numbers

- GPS integration for directions to provider locations

- Offline capability for essential crisis information

Student/Family-Friendly Versions

Professional resource databases often use language and categories that make sense to providers but confuse the families trying to use them. Create versions specifically designed for student and family users.

Family-friendly adaptations:

- Plain language descriptions that avoid clinical jargon

- Organization by common concerns ("My teenager is anxious," "My child won't go to school") rather than professional service categories

- Clear explanations of what different types of help involve

- Realistic timelines and expectations for accessing services
- Cost information presented in ways that help families plan and budget

Student-focused versions:

- Age-appropriate language and design
- Emphasis on confidentiality and student rights
- Information about accessing help independently when appropriate
- Peer support and online resources specifically for teenagers
- Clear explanations of what therapy and mental health services are actually like

Organization Strategies

How you organize resource information determines whether users can find what they need quickly or become frustrated and give up. Different users need different organizational approaches.

By Service Type

Organizing resources by the type of service provided helps users who know what kind of help they're looking for but need to find specific providers.

Service type categories:

- Crisis intervention and emergency services
- Individual therapy and counseling
- Family therapy and family support
- Psychiatric medication evaluation and management
- Specialized programs (eating disorders, substance abuse, trauma)

- Support groups and peer support
- Educational and advocacy services

Within each service category, organize by:

- Geographic location (closest to school/community first)
- Availability (shortest wait times first)
- Insurance acceptance (most commonly accepted insurance first)
- Special populations served (adolescent specialists first)

By Insurance Accepted

Many families' first question is "Do you take our insurance?" Organizing resources by insurance acceptance helps families quickly identify realistic options.

Insurance organization considerations:

- List major insurance plans operating in your area
- Include Medicaid and state insurance programs
- Create categories for sliding scale and reduced-fee services
- Identify providers who accept self-pay patients
- Include information about insurance verification processes

Insurance category design:

- Clear headings for each major insurance plan
- Cross-references when providers accept multiple insurance types
- Up-to-date information about insurance changes and updates
- Contact information for insurance verification

- Explanation of common insurance terms (copay, deductible, prior authorization)

By Age Served

Mental health services are often age-specific, and families need to know which providers actually work with their child's age group.

Age-based organization:

- Early childhood (ages 0-5)

- Elementary school age (ages 6-11)

- Middle school/early adolescence (ages 12-14)

- High school/late adolescence (ages 15-18)

- Transition age youth (ages 18-21)

- Family services (all ages)

Age considerations within categories:

- Providers who specialize in specific developmental stages

- Services that require different approaches for different ages

- Resources that serve multiple age groups vs. age-specific programs

- Transition planning resources for students aging out of services

By Language/Culture

Cultural and linguistic competency significantly affects the success of mental health treatment. Organizing resources by cultural and language capabilities helps families find appropriate matches.

Cultural organization considerations:

- Primary languages spoken by providers

- Cultural communities specifically served

- Religious or spiritual approaches to mental health

- Providers with experience with specific immigrant or refugee populations

- LGBTQ+ affirming providers

- Providers experienced with specific cultural mental health concerns

Cultural competency information to include:

- Languages spoken by providers (not just availability of interpreters)

- Cultural backgrounds and training of providers

- Experience with specific cultural mental health issues

- Understanding of cultural barriers to mental health treatment

- Ability to incorporate cultural strengths and resources into treatment

Maintenance Protocols

Resource information changes constantly – providers move, insurance acceptance changes, wait times fluctuate, and new services become available. Systematic maintenance protocols ensure your resource guides remain accurate and useful.

Quarterly Update Schedules

Regular updates prevent your resource database from becoming outdated and unreliable. Quarterly updates provide a good balance between staying current and manageable workload.

Quarterly update tasks:

- Contact high-use providers to verify contact information and services

- Check wait times and availability for key resources
- Verify insurance acceptance and payment options
- Update any changes in location, staff, or services
- Add new resources discovered since last update
- Remove resources that are no longer available or appropriate

Quarterly update process:

1. **Month 1:** Review and update crisis services and emergency resources

2. **Month 2:** Review and update outpatient therapy and medication management resources

3. **Month 3:** Review and update specialized services and support programs

4. **End of quarter:** Compile all updates and distribute revised resource guides

Accuracy Verification Systems

Systematic verification ensures that the information in your database is reliable and current. Inaccurate information damages your credibility and wastes families' time.

Verification protocols:

- Call every resource at least twice per year to confirm basic information
- Test websites and online resources for functionality
- Verify that services described are actually available
- Check that insurance and payment information is current
- Confirm that providers are still accepting new patients
- Update wait time information regularly

Verification documentation:

- Date of last verification contact
- Person who completed verification
- Changes made during verification
- Next scheduled verification date
- Notes about any concerns or issues discovered

Gap Analysis Procedures

Regular analysis of your resource database helps identify missing services and unmet needs in your community.

Gap analysis questions:

- What types of referrals do you receive most frequently?
- Which services have the longest wait times or highest demand?
- What populations are underserved by available resources?
- Where do families have to travel farthest to access needed services?
- Which insurance plans have limited provider options?
- What cultural or linguistic communities lack appropriate resources?

Using gap analysis results:

- Advocate with community organizations and funders for needed services
- Recruit new providers to fill identified gaps
- Develop partnerships to address unmet needs

- Share gap analysis results with community mental health coalitions

- Use data to support grant applications or funding requests

Creating Your Community Mental Health Safety Net

You've now learned how to systematically build, maintain, and organize a resource database that transforms your ability to connect students and families with appropriate mental health support. But the real value of this work goes beyond just having good information – it's about creating a safety net that ensures no student falls through the cracks because they couldn't access the help they needed.

Your resource database becomes a bridge between identification and intervention, between recognizing that a student needs help and ensuring they actually receive it. When you can immediately provide families with specific, accurate, actionable information about mental health resources, you dramatically increase the likelihood that they'll follow through and get the support their child needs.

The systematic approach outlined in this section – the 12-week implementation plan, the relationship-building strategies, the multiple format options, and the ongoing maintenance protocols – ensures that your resource system remains current, comprehensive, and genuinely useful to the families and students you serve.

Most importantly, building your resource database isn't a one-time project – it's an ongoing professional responsibility that strengthens your entire community's ability to support student mental health. The relationships you build with mental health providers, the partnerships you maintain, and the advocacy you engage in all contribute to a stronger system of care that benefits not just your current students, but future students and families as well.

The time and effort you invest in resource mapping pays dividends every time a family successfully connects with appropriate mental health support, every time a student gets help before a crisis occurs, and every time you can confidently say, "Yes, I know exactly who can help you with that."

Section 6: Navigating The System

Chapter 6.1: Understanding Your Legal Landscape

At 2:15 PM on a Tuesday, you receive a frantic call from the mother of 17-year-old Jason. "I just got off the phone with my son's therapist, and she says she can't tell me anything about his treatment because he's almost 18. But the school counselor said you've been coordinating his care and sharing information with his teachers. I don't understand – who can know what about my son's mental health, and what are my rights as his parent?"

Legal questions about student mental health create some of the most confusing and anxiety-provoking situations you'll face as a school nurse. The intersection of federal privacy laws, state regulations, professional ethics, and institutional policies creates a complex web that can feel impossible to navigate. Add the urgency of mental health crises, and you're often making critical decisions about information sharing and reporting requirements under pressure.

But here's the thing: understanding your legal landscape isn't just about avoiding lawsuits or staying out of trouble. It's about creating clear, ethical frameworks that actually improve your ability to help students and families. When you understand what information you can share, with whom, and under what circumstances, you can build more effective support systems while maintaining appropriate confidentiality protections.

FERPA vs. HIPAA Quick Guide

The confusion between FERPA (Family Educational Rights and Privacy Act) and HIPAA (Health Insurance Portability and Accountability Act) creates more problems for school nurses than almost any other legal issue. Most school staff have heard of both laws but don't understand when each applies or how they interact.

237

When Each Applies

FERPA applies to:

- Information maintained by schools and school districts

- Educational records that include personally identifiable information about students

- Any record that is maintained by the school and used for educational purposes

- Health records maintained by school personnel for educational purposes

- Mental health information collected by school staff as part of educational services

HIPAA applies to:

- Healthcare providers, health plans, and healthcare clearinghouses (called "covered entities")

- Healthcare information transmitted electronically

- Medical records maintained by healthcare professionals outside the school setting

- Mental health treatment records maintained by private practitioners

Here's where it gets tricky: School nurses exist in a unique position where both laws might apply to different aspects of your work, sometimes simultaneously.

Your work that falls under FERPA:

- Mental health screening results conducted as part of school health services

- Documentation of mental health interventions provided at school

- Coordination with teachers and school staff about student mental health needs

- Communication with parents about school-based mental health observations

- Records of how mental health concerns affect educational performance

Your work that might fall under HIPAA:

- If you're employed by a healthcare organization that contracts with the school

- When you're functioning as a healthcare provider independent of your school role

- If your school operates a school-based health center that provides medical services

- When coordinating with outside healthcare providers who are HIPAA-covered entities

Key Differences in School Settings

Understanding the practical differences between FERPA and HIPAA helps you make appropriate decisions about information sharing and documentation.

FERPA characteristics:

- Gives parents rights to access their child's educational records (until age 18)

- Allows sharing within the school for "legitimate educational interest"

- Requires written consent for sharing outside the school (with specific exceptions)

- Focuses on educational benefit and student success

- Allows students to access their own records at age 18 and control further sharing

HIPAA characteristics:

- Gives patients (or parents of minors) rights to access medical records

- Requires written authorization for most information sharing

- Has different rules for mental health information (often more restrictive)

- Focuses on medical treatment and healthcare operations

- Allows sharing for treatment, payment, and healthcare operations without consent

Practical implications for your daily work:

- Mental health information you gather at school is generally covered by FERPA, not HIPAA

- You can share FERPA-protected information with teachers and school staff who have legitimate educational interest

- Sharing with outside mental health providers requires different protocols depending on whether FERPA or HIPAA governs the interaction

- Documentation requirements differ between the two laws

Information Sharing Decision Tree

When you're unsure whether you can share mental health information, use this systematic approach:

Step 1: Identify what law governs the information

- Was this information collected in your role as school personnel? (Usually FERPA)

- Was this information created by outside healthcare providers? (Usually HIPAA)

- Are you sharing with school staff or outside parties?

Step 2: Determine the purpose of sharing

- Educational benefit for the student? (FERPA allows extensive sharing within school)

- Healthcare coordination? (May require consent under either law)

- Safety/emergency? (Both laws have emergency exceptions)

Step 3: Check consent requirements

- FERPA: Generally allows sharing within school without consent, requires consent for outside sharing

- HIPAA: Generally requires written authorization for sharing mental health information

Step 4: Document your decision-making process

- What information are you sharing and why?

- What legal authority allows this sharing?

- What safeguards are in place to protect privacy?

Common Misconceptions Clarified

Misconception #1: "HIPAA prevents us from sharing any health information" *Reality:* HIPAA rarely applies to school health records. Most school health information is protected by FERPA, which allows much more flexibility for educational purposes.

Misconception #2: "We can't tell teachers anything about student mental health" *Reality:* FERPA explicitly allows sharing educational records with school staff who have legitimate educational interest, including information about mental health concerns that affect educational performance.

Misconception #3: "Parents have absolute rights to their child's mental health information" *Reality:* While parents generally have strong rights under FERPA, there are exceptions for mature minors and situations where disclosure might harm the student.

Misconception #4: "Once students turn 18, parents have no rights to information" *Reality:* While FERPA rights transfer to students at 18, there are exceptions for emergency situations and when students are dependents for tax purposes.

Misconception #5: "We need written consent to share any mental health information" *Reality:* FERPA allows verbal consent for many purposes and has numerous exceptions that allow sharing without any consent.

Mandatory Reporting Requirements

Mandatory reporting laws create legal obligations for school nurses to report suspected abuse, neglect, or other harmful situations. Understanding these requirements protects both you and the students you serve.

State-Specific Requirements

Mandatory reporting requirements vary significantly by state, and you need to understand the specific laws in your jurisdiction.

Universal elements across all states:

- School personnel (including nurses) are mandated reporters in every state
- Reports must be made when you have reasonable suspicion of abuse or neglect
- Good faith reports are protected from liability

- Failure to report can result in criminal charges and professional consequences

State variations you need to research:

- Specific definition of "reasonable suspicion" in your state

- Which situations require reporting (all states require abuse/neglect reporting, but some require additional reporting)

- Timeline requirements for making reports

- Whether you need to inform parents before reporting

- Specific agency to receive reports

- Documentation requirements

Common mandatory reporting situations:

- Physical abuse by parents or caregivers

- Sexual abuse or exploitation

- Severe neglect affecting child's health or safety

- Emotional abuse (in states that include this)

- Child exposed to domestic violence (in some states)

- Self-harm that parents refuse to address (in some circumstances)

Mental health specific reporting considerations:

- When parents refuse emergency mental health treatment for suicidal child

- When family situation is contributing to mental health crisis

- When student reports abuse as factor in their mental health problems

- When mental health symptoms suggest possible abuse or neglect

Reporting Timeline Requirements

Every state has specific timelines for making mandatory reports, and failing to meet these timelines can have serious legal consequences.

Immediate reporting (within 24 hours or immediately):

- Most states for suspected child abuse
- Situations where child is in immediate danger
- Sexual abuse cases
- Severe physical abuse or neglect

48-72 hour reporting:

- Some states for less immediate abuse concerns
- Cases where safety planning can ensure immediate safety
- Situations requiring investigation but not emergency response

Mental health related timeline considerations:

- Mental health crises that suggest possible abuse require immediate reporting
- Chronic mental health problems related to family dysfunction may allow longer timelines
- When in doubt, err on the side of reporting sooner rather than later

Documentation Standards

Proper documentation protects you legally while ensuring that reported information is useful to investigating agencies.

Essential documentation elements:

- Date, time, and circumstances of disclosure or observation
- Exact words used by student (when possible)
- Objective description of physical signs or behaviors observed
- Who was present during disclosure or observation
- Actions taken and agencies notified
- Follow-up activities and timeline

Documentation standards:

- Use objective, factual language rather than interpretations or opinions
- Include specific details rather than general statements
- Document contemporaneously (as close to the event as possible)
- Maintain confidentiality of documentation
- Store documentation securely according to school policy

What TO document:

- Student's exact words about abuse or neglect
- Physical signs observed (bruises, injuries, hygiene issues)
- Behavioral indicators witnessed directly
- Student's emotional state during disclosure
- Safety measures implemented
- Reports made and to which agencies

What NOT to document:

- Your personal opinions about family dynamics
- Unverified information from other sources

- Speculation about what might have happened

- Judgmental language about parents or caregivers

- Information not directly related to safety concerns

Liability Protection Understanding

Understanding your legal protections helps you make appropriate reporting decisions without fear of personal legal consequences.

Legal protections for mandated reporters:

- Good faith immunity: You cannot be sued for making reports in good faith

- Criminal immunity: You cannot be charged criminally for making good faith reports

- Civil immunity: You are protected from lawsuits by families for making appropriate reports

- Employment protection: You cannot be fired or disciplined for making mandatory reports

Requirements for legal protection:

- Report must be made in good faith (honest belief that abuse or neglect occurred)

- Report must be made according to state law requirements and timelines

- Report must be made to appropriate agencies

- You must follow established procedures for making reports

Situations that might not be protected:

- Reports made maliciously or in bad faith

- Reports containing information you know to be false

- Failure to follow proper reporting procedures

- Sharing confidential information beyond what's required for reporting

When legal protection applies to mental health situations:

- Reporting family abuse that's contributing to student's mental health crisis

- Reporting parents' refusal to seek emergency mental health treatment

- Reporting situations where mental health symptoms suggest abuse or neglect

- Reporting threats made by family members against student with mental health problems

Chapter 6.2: Confidentiality Management

Managing confidentiality in school-based mental health work requires you to balance competing interests: students' rights to privacy, parents' rights to information about their children, educators' needs for information to support students effectively, and legal requirements for reporting and information sharing. Getting this balance right builds trust with students and families while ensuring appropriate collaboration and legal compliance.

Confidentiality in school settings is more complex than in traditional healthcare settings because schools serve multiple functions – educational, social, and increasingly, mental health support. Students often disclose sensitive information to school nurses, expecting privacy, while parents and teachers need enough information to provide appropriate support. Your challenge is creating confidentiality practices that protect privacy while facilitating effective help.

Age-Based Consent Guidelines

Understanding how consent and confidentiality rights change as students get older helps you make appropriate decisions about information sharing and treatment coordination.

Minor Consent Laws by State

State laws vary significantly regarding when minors can consent to their own mental health treatment and what confidentiality rights they have.

General categories of minor consent:

- **Emancipated minors:** Usually age 16+ who are legally independent (married, in military, living independently)

- **Mature minors:** Varies by state, usually 14-16+ who demonstrate capacity to make healthcare decisions

- **Emergency situations:** Most states allow minor consent for emergency mental health treatment

- **Specific conditions:** Some states allow minor consent for mental health, substance abuse, or reproductive health

State variations to research:

- Minimum age for mental health consent in your state

- Whether parental notification is required even when minors can consent

- Exceptions for emergency mental health treatment

- Rights of parents to access mental health records when minors consent to treatment

- School's role in minor consent for mental health services

Practical implications for school nurses:

- Students may have different confidentiality rights depending on their age and state laws

- Some students can consent to outside mental health treatment without parental involvement

- Your documentation and information sharing must account for students' legal rights

- Emergency mental health interventions may have different rules than ongoing treatment

Mature Minor Considerations

The mature minor doctrine recognizes that some younger students may have the capacity to make healthcare decisions even if they haven't reached the legal age of consent.

Factors in mature minor assessment:

- Student's age and mental capacity
- Complexity of the decision being made
- Student's understanding of risks and benefits
- Whether delay would increase risk to student
- Student's emotional maturity and stability
- Previous experience with healthcare decision-making

Mature minor applications in school mental health:

- 15-year-old with good insight requesting confidential counseling for family problems
- 16-year-old seeking information about mental health resources without parental involvement
- 14-year-old with depression who understands treatment options and wants therapy

Limitations of mature minor doctrine:

- Not recognized in all states or situations
- May not apply to major mental health interventions
- Doesn't override mandatory reporting requirements
- May not protect student from parental access to school records

Parent Access Rights

Understanding parents' rights to access their children's mental health information helps you balance family involvement with student privacy.

General parental rights under FERPA:

- Parents have rights to access their child's educational records until age 18

- This includes health records maintained by school personnel

- Parents can request meetings to discuss their child's mental health support at school

- Parents have rights to be notified about mental health policies and procedures

Limitations on parental access:

- Information that would endanger the student's safety

- Records where disclosure would violate other students' privacy

- Some states have exceptions for mature minors seeking mental health help

- Treatment records maintained by outside providers (covered by HIPAA, not FERPA)

Balancing parental rights with student privacy:

- Involve students in decisions about what to share with parents when appropriate

- Focus sharing on information parents need to support their child effectively

- Respect cultural and family values around privacy and mental health

- Use clinical judgment about when parental involvement helps or hinders treatment

Student Rights at 18

When students reach 18, their rights to control mental health information change significantly under FERPA.

Rights that transfer to students at 18:

- Right to access their own educational records
- Right to control who can access their records
- Right to request amendments to incorrect information
- Right to file complaints about privacy violations
- Right to provide or withhold consent for information sharing

Continued parental access exceptions:

- Students who are dependents for tax purposes
- Emergency situations where student cannot provide consent
- Students who provide written consent for parental access
- Some financial aid related information

Practical considerations for 18+ students:

- You need the student's consent, not parental consent, for information sharing
- Parents may still be involved if student consents or in emergencies
- Students control their own mental health treatment decisions
- Documentation and communication protocols change when students turn 18

Information Sharing Protocols

Clear protocols for sharing mental health information help you make consistent decisions that support students effectively while maintaining appropriate confidentiality protections.

Legitimate Educational Interest Standard

FERPA allows schools to share educational records, including mental health information, with school staff who have legitimate educational interest in the information.

Who has legitimate educational interest:

- Teachers who work directly with the student
- Counselors and social workers providing support
- Administrators involved in discipline or safety issues
- Special education staff if student receives those services
- Other school nurses or health staff
- Support staff who work directly with the student (aides, coaches, etc.)

What constitutes legitimate educational interest:

- Information needed to provide appropriate academic support
- Safety information that affects the student's school environment
- Behavioral strategies that help the student succeed academically
- Accommodation needs related to mental health conditions
- Crisis intervention and emergency response information

Information to share with legitimate educational interest:

- General nature of mental health concerns affecting school performance
- Specific accommodations or modifications needed
- Warning signs that indicate student needs additional support
- Crisis intervention strategies that work for the student

- Safety plans relevant to school environment

Information NOT to share even with legitimate educational interest:

- Detailed therapy session content
- Specific family dynamics not directly relevant to school
- Information about other family members' mental health
- Details about past trauma unless relevant to current school functioning

Team Communication Boundaries

Effective mental health support requires team coordination, but teams need clear boundaries about information sharing.

Core team members for mental health coordination:

- School nurse (often team coordinator)
- School counselor or social worker
- Relevant teachers and classroom staff
- Administrators when necessary
- Special education staff if applicable

Extended team members (as needed):

- Outside mental health providers (with consent)
- Parents and family members
- Medical providers
- Community support services

Boundaries for team communication:

- Share information on need-to-know basis for educational support

- Focus on school-relevant aspects of mental health concerns
- Respect student and family preferences about information sharing when possible
- Use secure communication methods for sensitive information
- Document team decisions about information sharing

Team communication protocols:

- Regular team meetings with structured agendas
- Secure written communication for ongoing coordination
- Clear designation of who communicates with outside providers
- Procedures for urgent information sharing between team members
- Documentation of team decisions and rationales

External Provider Coordination

Coordinating with outside mental health providers requires careful attention to consent requirements and information sharing agreements.

When coordination is beneficial:

- Ensuring consistency between school and therapeutic interventions
- Avoiding conflicting approaches to student's mental health needs
- Sharing observations that help providers understand student's functioning
- Coordinating crisis intervention and safety planning
- Supporting student's transition between different levels of care

Consent requirements for coordination:

- Written consent from parents (for students under 18)
- Written consent from students (for those 18 and over)
- Specific description of what information will be shared
- Clear timeframe for consent and sharing agreement
- Option for students/families to revoke consent

Information to share with outside providers (with consent):

- School-based observations of mental health symptoms
- Academic and social functioning at school
- Successful interventions and accommodations used at school
- Peer interactions and social dynamics
- Crisis incidents and effective responses

Information to request from outside providers:

- General treatment goals relevant to school functioning
- Recommendations for school-based support
- Warning signs to monitor for symptom changes
- Emergency protocols if student experiences crisis at school
- Expected timeline and goals for treatment

Emergency Exceptions

Both FERPA and state laws provide exceptions that allow information sharing without consent in emergency situations.

Emergency situations that allow information sharing:

- Immediate threat to student's life or safety
- Situations where student poses imminent danger to others

- Medical emergencies requiring immediate intervention

- Crisis situations where delay would significantly increase risk

- Situations requiring immediate family notification for safety reasons

Emergency information sharing protocols:

- Share only information necessary to address immediate safety concerns

- Document the emergency circumstances that justified sharing without consent

- Follow up with appropriate consent procedures when emergency resolves

- Limit sharing to individuals who need information to address emergency

- Review emergency sharing decisions to ensure they were appropriate

Post-emergency procedures:

- Obtain appropriate consent for ongoing information sharing

- Review emergency response to identify improvements needed

- Document lessons learned and policy implications

- Communicate with student and family about information shared during emergency

- Update safety plans based on emergency experience

Documentation Best Practices

Proper documentation protects students, families, and you while creating records that support effective mental health care coordination.

What to Document

Comprehensive documentation helps track student progress, supports continuity of care, and provides legal protection for your decisions.

Essential documentation elements:

- Date, time, and location of all mental health interactions
- Objective observations of student behavior and presentation
- Exact quotes from student when discussing mental health concerns
- Interventions provided and student response
- Referrals made and follow-up actions taken
- Communication with parents, teachers, and outside providers
- Safety assessments and planning activities

Mental health specific documentation:

- Screening tool results and interpretation
- Risk assessments for suicide, self-harm, or violence
- Crisis interventions and their effectiveness
- Medication side effects or concerns observed
- Academic and social functioning changes
- Family involvement and response to mental health concerns

Documentation timing:

- Document interactions as soon as possible after they occur
- Complete documentation within 24 hours of significant mental health events
- Update ongoing documentation regularly to reflect changes

- Document follow-up activities within reasonable timeframes

What Not to Write

Inappropriate documentation can create legal problems and damage therapeutic relationships with students and families.

Avoid documenting:

- Personal opinions about student's family or situation
- Speculation about causes of mental health problems
- Judgmental language about student, family, or other providers
- Information not directly relevant to student's school-based mental health needs
- Gossip or unverified information from other sources
- Your personal reactions or feelings about the situation

Inappropriate documentation examples:

- "Parents are clearly dysfunctional and causing student's problems"
- "Student is just seeking attention with these suicide threats"
- "Family probably has history of mental illness based on student's presentation"
- "I think the therapist doesn't know what they're doing"

Appropriate documentation alternatives:

- "Student reports family conflict affecting sleep and concentration"
- "Student continues to express suicidal thoughts despite safety planning"
- "Student's presentation suggests possible family stressors"

- "Coordination with outside therapist ongoing"

Storage Requirements

Proper storage of mental health documentation protects privacy while ensuring information is available when needed.

Physical storage requirements:

- Locked filing cabinets in secure areas
- Limited access to authorized personnel only
- Separation from general educational records when appropriate
- Protection from damage, loss, or unauthorized access
- Secure destruction procedures for outdated records

Electronic storage requirements:

- Password-protected systems with appropriate security measures
- Regular backups to prevent data loss
- Access logs to track who views mental health records
- Encryption for highly sensitive information
- Secure email and communication systems for sharing information

Access control procedures:

- Clear policies about who can access mental health documentation
- Training for staff with access about confidentiality requirements
- Regular review of access permissions and need for continued access

- Procedures for emergency access to records
- Documentation of who accesses records and when

Retention Timelines

Understanding how long to maintain mental health documentation helps you comply with legal requirements while managing storage needs.

General retention requirements:

- Follow your state's educational record retention requirements
- Maintain records longer if ongoing legal or clinical needs exist
- Consider student's continued enrollment and need for services
- Balance storage costs with legal and clinical needs
- Follow federal requirements for specific types of documentation

Common retention timelines:

- Active student mental health records: Maintained throughout enrollment
- Crisis intervention documentation: Often 3-7 years after graduation
- Referral documentation: May be shorter retention period
- Safety planning documentation: Usually maintained until student graduates
- Coordination records: Follow general educational record timelines

Destruction procedures:

- Use secure destruction methods for all mental health records
- Document destruction date and method used

261

- Ensure all copies (including electronic) are destroyed
- Consider legal holds that might prevent destruction
- Maintain log of destroyed records for audit purposes

Chapter 6.3: Re-integration Planning

Maria returns to school on a Wednesday morning after spending five days in a psychiatric hospital following a suicide attempt. Her parents are anxious about how she'll readjust to school, her teachers are unsure how to support her without making her feel different, and Maria herself is worried that everyone will know where she's been. Without a systematic re-integration plan, Maria might struggle to reconnect with her academic work, feel isolated from her peers, and potentially experience another mental health crisis.

Re-integration planning is one of your most important responsibilities as a school nurse, yet it's often overlooked in the urgency of managing mental health crises. Students who have been hospitalized for psychiatric reasons, participated in intensive outpatient programs, or taken extended time off for mental health treatment need deliberate, coordinated support to successfully return to the school environment.

Research shows that the first few weeks after mental health treatment are critical for long-term success. Students who receive structured re-integration support are significantly more likely to maintain treatment gains, continue their education successfully, and avoid future mental health crises. Without proper planning, students may face academic overwhelm, social isolation, or environments that trigger the same problems that led to their initial mental health crisis.

Post-Hospitalization Protocols

When students return from psychiatric hospitalization, they're often in a vulnerable state of recovery that requires careful coordination between hospital staff, school personnel, family members, and ongoing mental health providers.

48-Hour Contact Timeline

The first 48 hours after discharge are critical for preventing re-hospitalization and ensuring successful transition back to the school environment.

Within 24 hours of learning about discharge:

- Contact family to schedule re-entry meeting
- Communicate with hospital discharge planner if possible
- Alert core school team members about upcoming return
- Review student's previous accommodations and support plans
- Prepare temporary modifications for initial return period

Within 48 hours of student's return:

- Conduct comprehensive re-entry assessment
- Meet with student privately to discuss concerns and needs
- Implement initial safety and support measures
- Communicate with relevant teachers about student's return
- Schedule follow-up check-ins and support activities

Contact protocol priorities:

1. **Safety assessment:** Is student stable and safe to return to regular school environment?

2. **Support needs:** What accommodations or modifications are needed initially?

3. **Communication plan:** How will school, family, and providers coordinate?

4. **Timeline planning:** What does gradual re-integration look like for this student?

Information Gathering Checklist

Systematic information gathering ensures you understand the student's current status and needs without overwhelming them or their family.

Medical and psychiatric status:

- Current medications and potential side effects affecting school performance
- Activity restrictions or medical limitations
- Follow-up appointments and ongoing treatment plans
- Warning signs that might indicate worsening condition
- Emergency contacts and protocols if crisis occurs at school

Academic status assessment:

- Coursework missed during hospitalization
- Current capacity for academic demands
- Need for modified schedule or reduced course load
- Testing accommodations or alternative assessment needs
- Timeline for returning to full academic participation

Social and emotional readiness:

- Student's concerns about returning to school
- Peer relationship status and potential social challenges
- Comfort level with teachers and school staff knowing about hospitalization
- Coping strategies learned during treatment
- Family support and involvement in re-integration

Safety planning information:

- Triggers that might cause distress in school environment

265

- Effective coping strategies for school-specific stressors
- Preferred support people and safe spaces at school
- Early warning signs of symptom recurrence
- Crisis intervention preferences and protocols

Team Meeting Planning

Effective re-integration requires coordinated effort from multiple team members with clearly defined roles and responsibilities.

Core team members:

- School nurse (often team coordinator)
- Student's primary teachers or case manager
- School counselor or social worker
- Administrative representative
- Parents or guardians
- Student (when appropriate and desired)

Extended team members (as needed):

- Special education coordinator
- 504 plan coordinator
- Outside mental health providers
- Medical providers
- Peer support or mentors

Meeting agenda structure:

1. **Welcome and introductions** (establish supportive tone)
2. **Student status review** (current functioning and needs)

3. **Academic planning** (schedule modifications, accommodations, catch-up plans)

4. **Social support planning** (peer interactions, social activities)

5. **Safety planning** (crisis protocols, warning signs, intervention strategies)

6. **Communication protocols** (how team will stay coordinated)

7. **Timeline and follow-up** (check-in schedule, plan adjustments)

Meeting preparation:

- Schedule meeting promptly but allow student time to settle

- Ensure comfortable, private meeting space

- Prepare relevant documentation and assessment information

- Coordinate with outside providers if they're participating

- Create agenda that focuses on student's success and wellbeing

Safety Assessment Procedures

Re-entering school after psychiatric hospitalization requires ongoing safety assessment to ensure the environment supports continued recovery.

Initial safety assessment components:

- Current suicide risk level and protective factors

- Triggers specific to school environment

- Effectiveness of coping strategies in school setting

- Social stressors and peer relationship concerns

- Academic pressure tolerance and stress management

Ongoing safety monitoring:

- Daily informal check-ins during initial re-integration period

- Weekly formal assessments during first month

- Monthly follow-up meetings with core team

- Crisis response protocols specific to this student

- Communication with outside providers about school observations

Environmental safety modifications:

- Identify and modify potential triggers in school environment

- Create safe spaces student can access when feeling overwhelmed

- Establish clear protocols for when student needs support

- Train relevant staff in student-specific intervention strategies

- Develop communication systems for requesting help discreetly

Gradual Return Models

Most students benefit from gradual re-integration rather than immediate return to full academic schedules. Structured return models help students rebuild confidence and stamina while preventing overwhelm.

Week 1: Limited Attendance Plans

The first week focuses on getting students comfortable in the school environment while managing limited demands.

Typical Week 1 schedule:

- 2-4 hours per day maximum

- Focus on core academic subjects only

- Frequent check-ins with support staff

- Modified expectations for participation and assignments
- Flexible schedule allowing early dismissal if needed

Week 1 priorities:

- Rebuilding comfort with school environment
- Reconnecting with supportive teachers and staff
- Assessing academic readiness and capacity
- Identifying any immediate challenges or concerns
- Establishing routines and coping strategy use

Week 1 accommodations:

- Reduced course load or modified schedule
- Permission to leave class for support as needed
- Modified participation expectations
- No major tests or assignments due
- Additional time for adjustment without academic pressure

Support activities during Week 1:

- Daily check-ins with school nurse or counselor
- Brief meetings with each teacher to discuss needs
- Peer support introduction if appropriate
- Family communication about daily experiences
- Coordination with outside mental health providers

Week 2-3: Expanded Participation

Weeks 2-3 gradually increase academic demands while maintaining strong support structures.

Typical Week 2-3 progression:

- Increase to 4-6 hours per day
- Add back elective courses or additional subjects
- Begin modified assignment completion
- Introduce group work or social activities gradually
- Maintain regular support check-ins

Academic expectations Week 2-3:

- Modified assignments with reduced complexity or length
- Extended time for completing work
- Alternative assessment options when possible
- Gradual introduction of regular testing expectations
- Focus on participation and engagement over performance

Social integration Week 2-3:

- Gradual re-entry into lunch and social periods
- Participation in group activities with support
- Peer interaction monitoring and support
- Address social concerns or conflicts promptly
- Build positive peer connections and support networks

Monitoring and adjustment Week 2-3:

- Daily informal check-ins continue
- Weekly team meetings to assess progress
- Adjustment of plan based on student response
- Communication with family about home observations
- Coordination with mental health providers about treatment integration

Week 4+: Full Integration Strategies

By week 4, most students are ready to participate more fully in school activities while maintaining support systems.

Full integration goals:

- Return to regular schedule with accommodations as needed
- Resume full academic expectations with modifications
- Participate in extracurricular activities if desired
- Maintain peer relationships and social connections
- Use coping strategies independently in school environment

Ongoing support after full integration:

- Weekly check-ins with designated support person
- Monthly team meetings to review progress
- Continued accommodation implementation
- Crisis response protocols remain in place
- Regular communication with outside providers

Success indicators for full integration:

- Student attending school regularly without distress
- Academic performance improving or stabilizing
- Positive peer interactions and social connections
- Effective use of coping strategies when stressed
- Student reports feeling supported and successful at school

Progress Monitoring Systems

Systematic monitoring helps you track student progress and make timely adjustments to support plans.

Daily monitoring indicators:

- Attendance and punctuality patterns
- Mood and energy level observations
- Participation in classes and activities
- Social interactions with peers and staff
- Use of coping strategies and support services

Weekly assessment measures:

- Academic performance and assignment completion
- Social integration and peer relationships
- Mental health symptom stability
- Family feedback about home functioning
- Student self-report of adjustment and wellbeing

Monthly comprehensive review:

- Overall progress toward re-integration goals
- Effectiveness of current accommodations and support
- Need for plan modifications or additional services
- Coordination with outside mental health providers
- Planning for upcoming challenges or transitions

Academic Accommodations

Students returning from mental health treatment often need academic accommodations to support their continued recovery while maintaining educational progress.

504 Plan Considerations

Section 504 of the Rehabilitation Act provides important protections for students whose mental health conditions substantially limit major life activities.

Mental health conditions that may qualify for 504 plans:

- Depression that affects concentration, energy, or attendance
- Anxiety disorders that interfere with academic performance
- PTSD that impacts daily functioning at school
- Eating disorders affecting physical health and concentration
- Bipolar disorder requiring accommodation for mood episodes

Common 504 accommodations for mental health:

- Extended time on tests and assignments
- Alternative testing locations (quiet, private spaces)
- Modified attendance policies for mental health appointments
- Permission to leave class for brief breaks or support
- Reduced homework load during mental health episodes
- Alternative ways to demonstrate learning and knowledge

504 plan development process:

- Evaluation to determine substantial limitation in major life activity
- Team meeting including parents, student, and school personnel
- Development of specific accommodations based on individual needs
- Regular review and revision of plan as needed
- Coordination with mental health treatment when appropriate

Temporary Modifications

Not all students need formal 504 plans, but many benefit from temporary modifications during re-integration periods.

Academic modifications for re-integration:

- Reduced course load or modified schedule initially
- Extended deadlines for missed work during hospitalization
- Modified participation expectations during adjustment period
- Alternative formats for completing assignments
- Flexible attendance policies during initial return

Duration of temporary modifications:

- Usually 2-6 weeks depending on individual needs
- Regular review and adjustment based on student progress
- Gradual reduction of modifications as student stabilizes
- Transition to formal accommodations if long-term needs identified
- Documentation of modifications and their effectiveness

Make-up Work Management

Students returning from mental health treatment often face significant amounts of missed work that can feel overwhelming and trigger anxiety or depression.

Prioritizing make-up work:

- Focus on essential assignments and skills first
- Eliminate busy work or repetitive practice assignments
- Modify lengthy assignments to focus on key concepts
- Allow alternative ways to demonstrate understanding

274

- Provide extended timelines that don't create additional stress

Make-up work strategies:

- Break large assignments into smaller, manageable pieces
- Provide study guides or note summaries for missed content
- Offer tutoring or additional support for difficult concepts
- Allow collaboration with classmates for missed group work
- Consider partial credit for good faith efforts rather than perfect completion

Communication with teachers about make-up work:

- Clearly explain student's situation and needs (with appropriate consent)
- Provide specific guidelines about modified expectations
- Set reasonable timelines that support student success
- Regular check-ins about student progress and challenges
- Flexibility to adjust plans based on student response

Testing Accommodations

Students with mental health concerns often need modified testing arrangements to demonstrate their knowledge fairly.

Common testing accommodations:

- Extended time (typically 50-100% additional time)
- Alternative testing location (quiet, distraction-free environment)
- Frequent breaks during long tests
- Alternative test formats (oral vs. written, multiple choice vs. essay)

- Use of assistive technology or tools
- Testing at optimal times of day for individual student

Implementation of testing accommodations:

- Clear communication with all teachers about accommodation needs
- Coordination of testing schedules to avoid conflicts
- Training for staff administering accommodated tests
- Regular review of accommodation effectiveness
- Adjustment of accommodations based on changing needs

Success Monitoring

Effective re-integration requires ongoing monitoring that tracks progress, identifies challenges early, and allows for timely plan adjustments.

Daily Check-in Protocols

Regular, brief check-ins help maintain connection with students while monitoring their adjustment to school re-entry.

Daily check-in structure:

- 5-10 minute conversations at consistent times
- Focus on current day's experiences and challenges
- Assessment of mood, energy, and coping strategy use
- Identification of any immediate needs or concerns
- Planning for upcoming challenges or activities

Daily check-in questions:

- "How are you feeling about being back at school today?"
- "What's been the hardest part of your day so far?"

- "Have you used any of your coping strategies today?"

- "Is there anything you need help with right now?"

- "How are you feeling about tomorrow?"

Documentation of daily check-ins:

- Brief notes about student's mood and functioning

- Any concerns or challenges identified

- Coping strategies used and their effectiveness

- Support provided or referrals made

- Plans for follow-up or additional support

Warning Sign Identification

Early identification of warning signs helps prevent mental health crises and allows for prompt intervention.

Academic warning signs:

- Declining grades or assignment completion

- Increased absences or tardiness

- Difficulty concentrating or staying focused

- Avoidance of challenging tasks or activities

- Loss of interest in previously enjoyed subjects

Social warning signs:

- Withdrawal from friends or social activities

- Conflicts with peers or staff members

- Changes in social group or friend relationships

- Isolation during lunch or free time

- Avoiding group activities or collaborative work

Emotional/behavioral warning signs:

- Changes in mood, energy, or emotional regulation
- Increased anxiety or worry about school activities
- Return of symptoms that led to initial hospitalization
- Changes in sleep, appetite, or physical health
- Increased use of unhealthy coping strategies

Progress Communication

Regular communication with all stakeholders helps maintain coordination and allows for collaborative problem-solving.

Weekly progress updates:

- Brief reports to parents about school adjustment
- Communication with teachers about student functioning
- Coordination with outside mental health providers
- Documentation of progress toward re-integration goals
- Identification of needed plan adjustments

Monthly comprehensive reviews:

- Team meetings with all key stakeholders
- Formal assessment of accommodation effectiveness
- Planning for upcoming challenges or transitions
- Celebration of successes and progress made
- Revision of plans based on changing needs

Plan Adjustment Triggers

Knowing when to modify re-integration plans helps ensure they remain responsive to students' changing needs.

Triggers for plan acceleration:

- Student demonstrating greater capacity than expected
- Rapid improvement in functioning and adjustment
- Student requesting increased challenges or participation
- Strong family and peer support facilitating faster progress
- Effective coping strategy use and symptom management

Triggers for plan deceleration:

- Signs of increasing stress or symptom recurrence
- Academic or social challenges creating overwhelming pressure
- Family or outside provider concerns about pace of re-integration
- Student expressing need for more time or support
- Environmental factors creating additional stressors

Triggers for major plan revision:

- Significant changes in student's mental health status
- New information about learning needs or disabilities
- Changes in family situation or support system
- Feedback from outside providers about treatment goals
- Student's own insights about what works best for their success

---

Mastering Your Professional Framework

You now have the tools to navigate the complex legal and practical challenges of providing mental health support in school settings. Understanding FERPA vs. HIPAA, managing confidentiality appropriately, meeting mandatory reporting requirements, and planning effective re-integration creates a professional framework that protects both you and the students you serve.

But beyond legal compliance, these systems help you provide more effective mental health support. When you're confident about what information you can share and with whom, you can build stronger collaborative relationships with teachers, providers, and families. When you have clear re-integration protocols, students returning from mental health treatment have better outcomes and fewer setbacks.

The legal landscape around student mental health will continue to change as society's understanding of these issues develops. New privacy regulations, updated reporting requirements, and changing consent laws mean that staying informed about legal requirements is an ongoing professional responsibility.

Most importantly, your understanding of these systems allows you to focus on what matters most – helping students access the mental health support they need while maintaining appropriate ethical and legal standards. You're not just following rules; you're creating frameworks that facilitate healing, learning, and growth for the students and families you serve.

APPENDICES

Appendix A: Printable Assessment Tools

The assessment tools in this appendix provide you with ready-to-use forms that support systematic mental health screening and monitoring. These tools are designed to be printed, copied, and used directly with students in your school setting. Each tool includes clear instructions, scoring guidelines, and interpretation guidance to help you make informed decisions about student mental health needs.

ASQ Screening Forms (All Ages)

The Ask Suicide-Screening Questions (ASQ) toolkit provides validated screening forms specifically designed for different age groups. These forms are brief, evidence-based tools that help identify students who may be at risk for suicide.

ASQ for Ages 8-11 (Elementary Version)

Instructions: Ask these questions in a private setting. If the student answers "yes" to any question, follow your crisis intervention protocol immediately.

Screening Questions:

1. "In the past few weeks, have you wished you were dead?"

2. "In the past few weeks, have you felt that you or your family would be better off if you were dead?"

3. "In the past week, have you been having thoughts about killing yourself?"

4. "Have you ever tried to kill yourself?"

If ANY answer is "Yes":

- Do not leave student alone

- Implement immediate safety protocols

- Contact parents/guardians

- Arrange for emergency mental health evaluation

- Document exact responses and actions taken

ASQ for Ages 12+ (Adolescent Version)

Use the same four questions with age-appropriate follow-up based on responses.

Additional Assessment Questions for Positive Screens:

- "Can you tell me more about these thoughts?"

- "Have you thought about how you might hurt yourself?"

- "What has kept you safe so far?"

- "Who are the people you can talk to when you're struggling?"

Documentation Form:

Student Name: _____ Date: _____ Time: _____

Grade: _____ Age: _____ Screener: _____

ASQ Results:

□ Question 1: Yes / No

□ Question 2: Yes / No

□ Question 3: Yes / No

□ Question 4: Yes / No

If any "Yes" responses, immediate actions taken:

□ Student supervised continuously

□ Parents/guardians contacted at: _____

□ Crisis team activated

□ Emergency services contacted

□ Other: _____

Follow-up planned:

□ Same-day professional evaluation

□ Safety planning completed

□ Ongoing monitoring scheduled

□ Parent meeting scheduled for: _____

Student's exact words (if concerning):

_____

_____

Next review date: _____

PHQ-9 and GAD-7 (With Scoring Guides)

These validated screening tools help identify symptoms of depression and anxiety in students aged 12 and older.

PHQ-9 (Patient Health Questionnaire-9) for Adolescents

Instructions: Ask the student to think about the past two weeks when answering these questions.

Over the past 2 weeks, how often have you been bothered by any of the following problems?

Response options: 0 = Not at all, 1 = Several days, 2 = More than half the days, 3 = Nearly every day

1. Little interest or pleasure in doing things you usually enjoy

2. Feeling down, depressed, or hopeless

3. Trouble falling asleep, staying asleep, or sleeping too much

4. Feeling tired or having little energy

5. Poor appetite or overeating

6. Feeling bad about yourself or that you're a failure or have let yourself or your family down

7. Trouble concentrating on things like school work, reading, or watching TV

8. Moving or speaking so slowly that other people could have noticed, or being so fidgety or restless that you've been moving around a lot more than usual

9. Thoughts that you would be better off dead or thoughts of hurting yourself in some way

PHQ-9 Scoring Guide:

- **Total Score 0-4:** Minimal depression - Monitor, provide general mental health resources

- **Total Score 5-9:** Mild depression - Weekly check-ins, school counselor referral, parent notification

- **Total Score 10-14:** Moderate depression - Bi-weekly check-ins, professional referral recommended, parent meeting

- **Total Score 15-19:** Moderately severe depression - Daily monitoring, urgent professional referral, academic accommodations

- **Total Score 20-27:** Severe depression - Intensive monitoring, immediate professional evaluation, comprehensive support plan

Special attention to Question 9: ANY score other than 0 requires immediate suicide risk assessment using ASQ protocol.

GAD-7 (Generalized Anxiety Disorder-7)

Instructions: Ask about the past two weeks when answering these questions.

Over the past 2 weeks, how often have you been bothered by the following problems?

Response options: 0 = Not at all, 1 = Several days, 2 = More than half the days, 3 = Nearly every day

1. Feeling nervous, anxious, or on edge

2. Not being able to stop or control worrying

3. Worrying too much about different things

4. Trouble relaxing

5. Being so restless that it's hard to sit still

6. Becoming easily annoyed or irritable

7. Feeling afraid as if something awful might happen

GAD-7 Scoring Guide:

- **Total Score 0-4:** Minimal anxiety - Provide stress management resources, routine follow-up

- **Total Score 5-9:** Mild anxiety - Teach coping strategies, weekly check-ins, monitor for changes

- **Total Score 10-14:** Moderate anxiety - Counseling referral, academic accommodations, parent involvement

- **Total Score 15-21:** Severe anxiety - Immediate counseling referral, comprehensive support plan, possible medical evaluation

Elementary Behavior Checklists

For students in grades K-5, behavioral observations often provide more reliable information than self-report measures.

Elementary Mental Health Observation Checklist

Instructions: Check behaviors observed over the past 2 weeks. Focus on changes from student's typical behavior.

Emotional Indicators: □ Frequent crying or tearfulness □ Extreme mood swings □ Persistent sadness or flat affect □ Excessive worry or fearfulness □ Inappropriate emotional responses □ Explosive anger or tantrums □ Withdrawn or isolated behavior

Behavioral Indicators: □ Significant changes in activity level □ Sleep problems (tired, reports nightmares) □ Appetite changes (not eating, always hungry) □ Regression behaviors (thumb sucking, baby talk) □ Increased clinginess to adults □ Aggressive behavior toward peers or adults □ Self-soothing behaviors (rocking, repetitive actions)

Academic/Social Indicators: □ Decline in academic performance □ Difficulty concentrating or completing tasks □ Loss of interest in previously enjoyed activities □ Social withdrawal from peers □ Conflicts with friends □ Reluctance to participate in group activities □ Frequent requests to go home

Physical Indicators: □ Frequent complaints of headaches or stomachaches □ Changes in personal hygiene □ Unexplained injuries or marks □ Frequent bathroom requests □ Motor restlessness or inability to sit still □ Appears tired or lethargic

Scoring:

- **1-3 items checked:** Monitor, provide extra support

- **4-6 items checked:** Parent contact, counselor referral

- **7+ items checked:** Urgent parent meeting, professional evaluation recommended

Daily Mood Tracking Sheets

These tools help students and staff monitor mood patterns and identify triggers or improvements over time.

Student Daily Mood Tracker (Ages 8+)

Instructions: Complete this each day at the same time. Rate how you felt for most of the day.

Name: _____ Week of: _____

Mon Tue Wed Thu Fri Sat Sun

Mood Rating (1-10): ___ ___ ___ ___ ___ ___ ___

(1=very sad, 10=very happy)

Energy Level (1-10): ___ ___ ___ ___ ___ ___ ___

(1=no energy, 10=lots of energy)

Anxiety Level (1-10): ___ ___ ___ ___ ___ ___ ___

(1=very calm, 10=very anxious)

Sleep Quality:

□ Good □ Okay □ Poor □ Good □ Okay □ Poor [repeat for each day]

What helped you feel better today?

Mon: _____

Tue: _____

Wed: _____

Thu: _____

Fri: _____

What was most stressful today?

Mon: _____

Tue: _____

Wed: _____

Thu: _____

Fri: _____

Staff Observation Daily Tracker

Instructions: Complete brief observations for students on monitoring list.

Student: _____ Week of: _____ Observer: _____

Daily Observations:

Monday:

Mood/Energy: □ Good □ Fair □ Poor □ Concerning

Participation: □ Active □ Moderate □ Minimal □ Withdrawn

Social: □ Engaged □ Some interaction □ Isolated □ Conflicts

Notes: _____

[Repeat format for Tuesday-Friday]

Weekly Summary:

Patterns noticed: _____

Improvements: _____

Concerns: _____

Recommended actions: _____

Crisis Assessment Forms

Comprehensive forms for documenting crisis situations and safety planning.

Crisis Assessment Documentation Form

CONFIDENTIAL - MENTAL HEALTH CRISIS ASSESSMENT

Student Information:

Name: _____ DOB: _____ Grade: _____ Date: _____

Time crisis began: _____ Staff involved: _____

Location of incident: _____

Nature of Crisis:

□ Suicidal thoughts/statements □ Self-harm behavior

□ Aggressive behavior   □ Panic attack

□ Psychotic symptoms   □ Severe depression/withdrawal

□ Substance use   □ Other: _____

Immediate Safety Assessment:

Current risk level: □ Low □ Moderate □ High □ Imminent danger

Specific statements made:

_____

_____

Behaviors observed:

_____

_____

Precipitating events/triggers:

_____

Immediate Actions Taken:

□ Student continuously supervised

□ Safe environment provided

□ Crisis team activated at: _____

□ Parents contacted at: _____ Response: _____

□ Emergency services called at: _____

□ Medical evaluation arranged

□ Safety plan developed

□ Other: _____

Resources/Support Activated:

□ School counselor   □ School psychologist

□ Administration   □ Outside mental health provider

□ Medical provider   □ Emergency services

□ Other: _____

Follow-up Plan:

□ Professional evaluation scheduled for: _____

□ Daily check-ins assigned to: _____

□ Parent meeting scheduled for: _____

□ Academic accommodations needed

□ Ongoing safety monitoring

□ Other: _____

Assessment completed by: _____ Date: _____

Reviewed with supervisor: _____ Date: _____

Next review scheduled: _____

Appendix B: Parent Communication Materials

Effective communication with parents about mental health requires prepared materials that provide clear information while maintaining a supportive, non-judgmental tone.

Mental Health Screening Introduction Letters

English Version

Dear Parents and Guardians,

As part of our commitment to supporting the whole child, [School Name] is implementing routine mental health screening for all students. Just as we regularly check students' vision and hearing, we now recognize the importance of monitoring emotional wellness as part of comprehensive health care.

What is mental health screening?

Mental health screening involves brief, confidential questions about mood, stress, and emotional well-being. These screenings help us identify students who might benefit from additional support before small concerns become bigger problems.

What does screening involve?

- Brief questionnaires appropriate for your child's age

- Individual conversations with our school nurse or counselor

- Observation of social and academic functioning

- Coordination with you about any concerns identified

Your rights and your child's privacy:

- You may opt your child out of screening by contacting our office

- Results are kept confidential and used only for educational support

- We will contact you if screening suggests your child needs additional help

- You have the right to access any health records we maintain about your child

How screening helps:

- Early identification leads to better outcomes

- Students receive support before crises occur

- Families get connected with appropriate resources

- School staff can provide better educational support

What happens next?

If screening suggests your child would benefit from additional support, we will:

- Contact you to discuss our observations

- Provide information about available resources

- Help coordinate appropriate services

- Work with you to support your child's success at school

We believe that addressing mental health is just as important as addressing physical health. Our goal is to support every student's success by ensuring they have the emotional tools they need to learn and grow.

If you have questions about our mental health screening program, please contact:

[Name, Title, Phone, Email]

Thank you for partnering with us to support your child's complete well-being.

Sincerely,

[School Administrator Name and Title]

Spanish Version

Estimados Padres y Tutores,

Como parte de nuestro compromiso de apoyar al niño completo, [Nombre de la Escuela] está implementando evaluaciones rutinarias de salud mental para todos los estudiantes. Así como regularmente revisamos la vista y el oído de los estudiantes, ahora reconocemos la importancia de monitorear el bienestar emocional como parte del cuidado integral de la salud.

¿Qué es la evaluación de salud mental?

La evaluación de salud mental incluye preguntas breves y confidenciales sobre el estado de ánimo, el estrés y el bienestar emocional. Estas evaluaciones nos ayudan a identificar estudiantes que podrían beneficiarse de apoyo adicional antes de que las pequeñas preocupaciones se conviertan en problemas más grandes.

¿Qué incluye la evaluación?

- Cuestionarios breves apropiados para la edad de su hijo/a

- Conversaciones individuales con nuestra enfermera escolar o consejero

- Observación del funcionamiento social y académico

- Coordinación con usted sobre cualquier preocupación identificada

Sus derechos y la privacidad de su hijo/a:

- Puede excluir a su hijo/a de la evaluación contactando nuestra oficina

- Los resultados se mantienen confidenciales y se usan solo para apoyo educativo

- Le contactaremos si la evaluación sugiere que su hijo/a necesita ayuda adicional

- Tiene el derecho de acceder a cualquier registro de salud que mantengamos sobre su hijo/a

Cómo ayuda la evaluación:

- La identificación temprana conduce a mejores resultados

- Los estudiantes reciben apoyo antes de que ocurran crisis

- Las familias se conectan con recursos apropiados

- El personal escolar puede proporcionar mejor apoyo educativo

¿Qué pasa después?

Si la evaluación sugiere que su hijo/a se beneficiaría de apoyo adicional, nosotros:

- Le contactaremos para discutir nuestras observaciones

- Proporcionaremos información sobre recursos disponibles

- Ayudaremos a coordinar servicios apropiados

- Trabajaremos con usted para apoyar el éxito de su hijo/a en la escuela

Creemos que abordar la salud mental es tan importante como abordar la salud física. Nuestro objetivo es apoyar el éxito de cada estudiante asegurándonos de que tengan las herramientas emocionales que necesitan para aprender y crecer.

Si tiene preguntas sobre nuestro programa de evaluación de salud mental, por favor contacte:

[Nombre, Título, Teléfono, Email]

Gracias por asociarse con nosotros para apoyar el bienestar completo de su hijo/a.

Sinceramente,

[Nombre y Título del Administrador Escolar]

Resource List Templates

Community Mental Health Resources Template

MENTAL HEALTH RESOURCES FOR FAMILIES

[School Name] - [Date]

CRISIS RESOURCES (Available 24/7)

National Suicide Prevention Lifeline: 988

Crisis Text Line: Text HOME to 741741

[Local Crisis Hotline]: [Phone Number]

[Local Mobile Crisis Team]: [Phone Number]

Emergency Services: 911

OUTPATIENT MENTAL HEALTH SERVICES

[Organization Name]

Services: Individual therapy, family therapy, group therapy

Ages Served: Children, adolescents, adults

Insurance Accepted: [List major plans]

Languages: English, Spanish, [others]

Contact: [Phone] [Website]

Wait Time: Approximately [timeframe]

Location: [Address]

[Organization Name]

Services: Psychiatric evaluation, medication management

Ages Served: [Age ranges]

Insurance Accepted: [List major plans]

Contact: [Phone] [Website]

Wait Time: Approximately [timeframe]

Special Notes: [Specializations, requirements]

SPECIALIZED SERVICES

Eating Disorders:

[Organization Name] - [Phone] - [Services offered]

[Organization Name] - [Phone] - [Services offered]

Substance Abuse Treatment:

[Organization Name] - [Phone] - [Services offered]

[Organization Name] - [Phone] - [Services offered]

SUPPORT GROUPS

For Parents:

NAMI [Local Chapter] - [Meeting times/location] - [Phone]

[Local Parent Support Group] - [Details]

For Students:

[Teen Support Groups] - [Details]

[Peer Support Programs] - [Details]

FINANCIAL ASSISTANCE

[Community Mental Health Center] - Sliding scale fees

[Charitable Organization] - Treatment scholarships

[Insurance Navigation Program] - Help with coverage questions

EDUCATIONAL SUPPORT

[Learning Disability Services] - [Phone]

[Educational Advocates] - [Phone]

[Tutoring Services with Mental Health Focus] - [Phone]

HOW TO ACCESS SERVICES

1. Contact the provider directly to inquire about services

2. Ask about wait times and insurance acceptance

3. Request information about their experience with your child's age group

4. Inquire about culturally competent services if relevant

5. Ask about emergency contact procedures

QUESTIONS TO ASK PROVIDERS

- What is your experience working with [child's age group]?

- What approaches do you use for [specific concern]?

- How do you involve families in treatment?

- What should we expect from the first few sessions?

- How do you coordinate with schools?

- What are your emergency contact procedures?

For questions about these resources or help navigating services, contact:

[School Contact Name, Phone, Email]

This list is updated [frequency]. For the most current information, please verify details directly with providers.

Crisis Response Parent Guides

When Your Child is Having a Mental Health Crisis: A Guide for Parents

IMMEDIATE SAFETY STEPS

If your child is threatening suicide or self-harm:

1. Stay calm and don't leave them alone

2. Remove any means of harm (medications, sharp objects, etc.)

3. Listen without judging or trying to fix everything immediately

4. Call 988 (Suicide & Crisis Lifeline) for immediate guidance

5. Take them to the emergency room if they're in immediate danger

6. Contact their mental health provider if they have one

If your child is having a panic attack:

1. Stay with them in a calm, quiet space

2. Help them focus on slow, deep breathing

3. Remind them that panic attacks are temporary and will pass

4. Don't tell them to "just calm down" - validate that this is scary

5. After the attack passes, talk about what triggered it

6. Follow up with their healthcare provider

If your child is displaying aggressive behavior:

1. Ensure everyone's physical safety first

2. Stay calm and speak in a low, steady voice

3. Give them space and don't corner them

4. Remove other family members from the immediate area

5. Call 911 if anyone is in physical danger

6. Seek professional help to develop better coping strategies

WHAT TO EXPECT AT THE EMERGENCY ROOM

- Screening questions about safety and mental state

- Possible wait times that can be lengthy

- Evaluation by mental health professionals

- Discussion of safety planning and discharge options

- Referrals for ongoing mental health treatment

- Possible admission if safety concerns are severe

SUPPORTING YOUR CHILD AFTER A CRISIS

- Maintain routines as much as possible

- Don't treat them like they're fragile or broken

- Follow through on professional recommendations

- Communicate regularly with school staff

- Monitor for warning signs of future crises

- Take care of your own mental health too

COMMUNICATING WITH SCHOOL

What to share:

- That your child experienced a mental health crisis

- Any safety plans or strategies that work at home

- Medications or treatment changes that might affect school

- Your child's comfort level with teachers knowing about the situation

What schools can provide:

- Academic accommodations during recovery period

- Counseling and emotional support during school hours

- Coordination with outside mental health providers

- Crisis intervention if symptoms occur at school

LONG-TERM RECOVERY SUPPORT

- Consistent mental health treatment (therapy, medication management)

- Regular communication between home, school, and providers

- Development of coping strategies and crisis prevention skills

- Family therapy or parent support groups

- Patience with the recovery process - healing takes time

RESOURCES FOR PARENTS

National Alliance on Mental Illness (NAMI): 1-800-950-6264

Family-to-Family Support Programs: [Local contact information]

Crisis Text Line for Parents: Text HOME to 741741

[Local Parent Support Groups]: [Meeting information]

WARNING SIGNS TO WATCH FOR

- Talking about death or suicide

- Giving away possessions

- Sudden improvement after depression (may indicate decision to attempt suicide)

- Increased substance use

- Withdrawing from family and friends

- Changes in sleep, appetite, or personal hygiene

- Decline in academic performance

- Loss of interest in activities they usually enjoy

WHEN TO SEEK IMMEDIATE HELP

- Any mention of suicide or self-harm

- Aggressive behavior that threatens safety

- Signs of psychosis (hallucinations, delusions, extreme confusion)

- Severe panic attacks that don't respond to usual interventions

- Substance use combined with mental health crisis

- Any situation where you're concerned about immediate safety

Remember: Mental health crises are temporary, and with appropriate support, your child can recover and develop better coping skills for the future.

For immediate crisis support: 988 (Suicide & Crisis Lifeline)

For school-related questions: [School contact information]

Medication Information Sheets

Understanding Psychiatric Medications for Children and Adolescents

COMMON TYPES OF PSYCHIATRIC MEDICATIONS

ANTIDEPRESSANTS

Examples: Fluoxetine (Prozac), Sertraline (Zoloft), Escitalopram (Lexapro)

What they treat:

- Depression

- Anxiety disorders

- Obsessive-compulsive disorder

- Post-traumatic stress disorder

How they work:

- Adjust brain chemicals (neurotransmitters) that affect mood

- Usually take 4-6 weeks to see full effects

- May cause temporary side effects while body adjusts

Common side effects:

- Nausea or stomach upset (usually temporary)

- Changes in sleep patterns

- Headaches

- Changes in appetite

- Restlessness or agitation (especially in first few weeks)

What to monitor:
- Mood changes, especially in first few months

- Sleep and appetite patterns

- Academic performance and concentration

- Social interactions and behavior

ANTI-ANXIETY MEDICATIONS

Examples: Short-term medications like lorazepam; longer-term like buspirone

What they treat:
- Severe anxiety that interferes with daily functioning

- Panic attacks

- Specific phobias affecting school attendance

Important considerations:
- Often used short-term while learning coping strategies

- Some can be habit-forming and require careful monitoring

- Usually combined with therapy for best results

MOOD STABILIZERS

Examples: Lithium, Lamotrigine (Lamictal), Divalproex (Depakote)

What they treat:

- Bipolar disorder

- Severe mood swings

- Some cases of aggressive behavior

Monitoring requirements:

- Regular blood tests to check medication levels

- Monitoring for side effects affecting thinking or coordination

- Coordination between prescriber and school nurse

STIMULANT MEDICATIONS

Examples: Methylphenidate (Ritalin, Concerta), Amphetamine (Adderall, Vyvanse)

What they treat:

- ADHD symptoms

- Sometimes used for depression that doesn't respond to other treatments

School considerations:

- Often given in morning before school

- May affect appetite and lunch eating

- Can improve focus and academic performance

- May need afternoon doses administered at school

ANTIPSYCHOTIC MEDICATIONS

Examples: Risperidone (Risperdal), Aripiprazole (Abilify), Quetiapine (Seroquel)

What they treat:

- Psychotic disorders

- Severe behavioral problems

- Sometimes used for mood stabilization

- Autism-related behavioral concerns

Important side effects to monitor:

- Weight gain and metabolic changes

- Movement side effects (tremor, stiffness)

- Sedation affecting school performance

- Changes in hormone levels

WORKING WITH YOUR CHILD'S PRESCRIBER

Questions to ask:

- What specific symptoms is this medication targeting?

310

- How long before we see benefits?

- What side effects should we watch for?

- How will we know if the medication is working?

- What happens if my child misses a dose?

- Are there any foods, activities, or other medications to avoid?

- How often will you monitor my child's response?

Information to provide:

- Complete list of all medications and supplements

- Family history of mental health and medication responses

- Any previous medication trials and their results

- Your child's daily schedule and school demands

- Any concerns about side effects or effectiveness

SCHOOL COORDINATION

Share with school nurse:

- Medication name and dosing schedule

- Expected benefits and timeline

- Side effects that might affect school performance

- Emergency contact information for prescriber

- Any special instructions for medication administration

School can monitor:

- Academic performance and concentration

- Social interactions and peer relationships

- Physical symptoms during school hours

- Behavioral changes throughout the day

- Effectiveness of medication timing

MEDICATION SAFETY

Storage:

- Keep medications in original bottles with labels

- Store in secure location away from other children

- Don't store in hot cars or humid bathrooms

- Check expiration dates regularly

Administration:

- Give exactly as prescribed - don't skip doses or adjust amounts

- Use medication reminder systems if helpful

- Don't stop medications suddenly without prescriber guidance

- Keep backup supply for school if doses are given there

Emergency situations:

- Know signs of serious side effects requiring immediate medical attention

- Have emergency contact information for prescriber readily available

- Understand what to do if overdose is suspected

- Know which side effects require stopping medication immediately

SUPPORTING YOUR CHILD

- Explain medications in age-appropriate terms

- Emphasize that medications are tools to help them feel better

- Don't make them feel ashamed about needing medication

- Involve them in monitoring how they're feeling

- Encourage them to report side effects or concerns

- Celebrate improvements and progress

MEDICATION IS JUST ONE PART OF TREATMENT

Most effective treatment includes:

- Regular therapy or counseling

- Family support and involvement

- School accommodations when needed

- Healthy lifestyle habits (sleep, exercise, nutrition)

- Stress management and coping skills

- Regular monitoring by healthcare providers

Remember: Finding the right medication often takes time. Work closely with your child's healthcare team and don't hesitate to ask questions or report concerns.

For questions about school-related medication issues, contact:

[School Nurse Name and Contact Information]

Insurance Navigation Guides

Navigating Mental Health Insurance Coverage: A Parent's Guide

UNDERSTANDING YOUR MENTAL HEALTH BENEFITS

Key Terms to Know:

- Copay: Fixed amount you pay for each visit

- Deductible: Amount you pay before insurance starts covering costs

- Coinsurance: Percentage of costs you pay after meeting deductible

- Out-of-pocket maximum: Most you'll pay in a year

- In-network: Providers who accept your insurance plan

- Out-of-network: Providers who don't have contracts with your insurance

BEFORE YOU START LOOKING FOR PROVIDERS

Contact your insurance company to ask:

1. Do I need a referral from my primary care doctor for mental health services?

2. What is my copay for mental health visits?

3. Does my plan have a separate deductible for mental health?

4. How many therapy sessions are covered per year?

5. Which mental health providers in our area are in-network?

6. What's the difference in coverage between in-network and out-of-network?

7. Is prior authorization required for certain types of mental health treatment?

8. Does my plan cover psychological testing or evaluations?

FINDING IN-NETWORK PROVIDERS

Your insurance website should have:

- Provider directory searchable by location and specialty
- Information about whether providers are accepting new patients
- Contact information and basic credentials

When calling providers, ask:

- Do you accept [your specific insurance plan]?
- Are you currently accepting new patients?
- What is the current wait time for new appointments?
- Do you specialize in working with [your child's age group]?
- What approaches do you use for [specific mental health concern]?

UNDERSTANDING AUTHORIZATION REQUIREMENTS

Some insurance plans require:

- Referral from primary care doctor before seeing mental health providers

- Prior authorization for certain types of therapy

- Pre-approval for intensive services or longer-term treatment

- Regular reviews to continue coverage for ongoing therapy

Get authorizations in writing and keep copies for your records.

MAXIMIZING YOUR BENEFITS

- Use in-network providers whenever possible

- Understand your annual limits and plan accordingly

- Keep detailed records of all appointments and payments

- Ask about sliding scale fees if you're having financial difficulties

- Consider Employee Assistance Programs (EAP) if available through work

WHAT TO DO IF SERVICES ARE DENIED

1. Understand the reason for denial

2. Work with your provider to submit additional information if needed

3. File an appeal if you believe the denial is incorrect

4. Contact your state insurance commissioner if appeals are unsuccessful

5. Consider external review processes if available

PAYING FOR OUT-OF-NETWORK SERVICES

If you choose an out-of-network provider:

- Understand your out-of-network benefits (usually much lower coverage)

- Ask provider about payment plans or sliding scale fees

- Keep detailed receipts for potential reimbursement

- Submit claims promptly according to your plan's requirements

- Consider using Health Savings Account (HSA) or Flexible Spending Account (FSA) funds

ALTERNATIVES WHEN INSURANCE DOESN'T COVER ENOUGH

Community mental health centers:

- Often provide sliding scale fees based on income

- May have shorter wait times than private providers

- Usually accept Medicaid and have experience with insurance issues

University training clinics:

- Supervised therapy students provide services at reduced cost

- Often high-quality care with close supervision

- May have specialized programs for children and adolescents

School-based services:

- Counseling and support services at no cost to families

- Convenient access during school hours

- Coordination with academic support

Online therapy platforms:

- Often less expensive than traditional therapy

- May be covered by some insurance plans

- Good option for ongoing support between in-person sessions

KEEPING TRACK OF YOUR MENTAL HEALTH EXPENSES

Create a simple tracking system:

- Date of service

- Provider name

- Type of service

- Amount charged

- Insurance payment

- Your out-of-pocket cost

- Remaining benefits for the year

This helps you:

- Monitor your progress toward deductible and out-of-pocket maximum

- Track remaining covered sessions

- Prepare for insurance appeals if needed

- Budget for ongoing mental health expenses

SPECIAL CONSIDERATIONS FOR CHILDREN

- Some providers specialize in pediatric mental health and may be worth out-of-network costs

- Ask about family therapy benefits - sometimes covered differently than individual therapy

- Understand coverage for psychological testing often needed for school accommodations

- Consider how insurance changes (job changes, etc.) might affect ongoing treatment

ADVOCACY AND APPEALS

If insurance denies coverage:

1. Request written explanation of denial

2. Review your plan documents to understand your benefits

3. Work with provider's office - they often have experience with appeals

4. Submit additional documentation if requested

5. Use your plan's formal appeal process

6. Contact your employer's HR department if you have workplace insurance

7. Seek help from patient advocacy organizations if needed

QUESTIONS TO ASK YOUR EMPLOYER

If you have workplace insurance:

- Are there mental health benefits beyond what's in the standard plan?

- Do we have an Employee Assistance Program (EAP) that provides free counseling?

- Are there wellness programs that might help with mental health?

- Can I change plans during open enrollment to better cover mental health needs?

EMERGENCY MENTAL HEALTH SERVICES

Important: Emergency mental health services are typically covered even if you go out-of-network, but confirm this with your insurance company.

- Emergency room visits for mental health crises

- Crisis intervention services

- Involuntary psychiatric hospitalization

- Mobile crisis team responses

Always follow up with your insurance company after emergency services to understand coverage and next steps.

FOR MORE HELP WITH INSURANCE ISSUES

- Your state's insurance commissioner's office

- Patient advocate organizations

- Mental Health America local chapters

- NAMI (National Alliance on Mental Illness) local chapters

- Healthcare.gov resources and consumer assistance

Remember: Insurance navigation can be frustrating, but mental health coverage has improved significantly in recent years. Don't let insurance barriers prevent your child from getting needed mental health support.

For questions about school-based mental health services that don't require insurance, contact:

[School Contact Information]

Appendix C: Quick Reference Guides

These laminated reference cards and posters provide essential information that you need to access quickly during busy school days.

Psychotropic Medication Side Effects Chart

QUICK REFERENCE: MEDICATION SIDE EFFECTS TO MONITOR AT SCHOOL

ANTIDEPRESSANTS (SSRIs)

Common: Fluoxetine (Prozac), Sertraline (Zoloft), Escitalopram (Lexapro)

Monitor for:

✓ Initial activation/agitation (first 2-4 weeks)

✓ Changes in sleep patterns

✓ Appetite changes affecting lunch eating

✓ Headaches or nausea

✓ Restlessness or fidgeting

✓ Social disinhibition (saying inappropriate things)

RED FLAGS:

• Increased suicidal thoughts (especially weeks 1-4)

- Manic symptoms (excessive energy, pressured speech)

- Severe agitation or aggression

STIMULANTS

Common: Methylphenidate (Ritalin, Concerta), Amphetamine (Adderall, Vyvanse)

Monitor for:

√ Appetite suppression (not eating lunch)

√ Sleep difficulties affecting next-day performance

√ Growth changes over time

√ Mood changes when medication wears off ("rebound")

√ Tics or repetitive movements

√ Social withdrawal or personality changes

RED FLAGS:

- Chest pain or rapid heart rate

- Hallucinations or paranoid thoughts

- Severe mood swings or aggression

- Signs of medication misuse

MOOD STABILIZERS

Common: Lithium, Lamotrigine (Lamictal), Divalproex (Depakote)

Monitor for:

✓ Drowsiness affecting academic performance

✓ Tremor or coordination problems

✓ Confusion or memory problems

✓ Weight gain over time

✓ Increased thirst or urination

✓ Nausea or stomach upset

RED FLAGS:

• Severe rash (especially with Lamictal)

• Signs of lithium toxicity (confusion, tremor, coordination problems)

• Severe sedation or cognitive impairment

ANTIPSYCHOTICS

Common: Risperidone (Risperdal), Aripiprazole (Abilify), Quetiapine (Seroquel)

Monitor for:

✓ Sedation affecting school performance

✓ Weight gain and increased appetite

✓ Movement side effects (tremor, stiffness, restlessness)

✓ Dizziness when standing up quickly

✓ Difficulty regulating body temperature

✓ Changes in social interaction

RED FLAGS:

• Severe movement side effects (dystonia, tardive dyskinesia)

• High fever with confusion (neuroleptic malignant syndrome)

• Significant metabolic changes

• Severe sedation affecting safety

ANTI-ANXIETY MEDICATIONS

Common: Lorazepam (Ativan), Clonazepam (Klonopin), Buspirone (Buspar)

Monitor for:

✓ Drowsiness affecting academic performance

✓ Confusion or memory problems

✓ Coordination difficulties

✓ Paradoxical reactions (increased agitation)

✓ Withdrawal symptoms if doses missed

RED FLAGS:

• Severe respiratory depression

• Signs of tolerance or dependence

• Dangerous interactions with other substances

WHEN TO CONTACT PRESCRIBER IMMEDIATELY:

• Any thoughts of self-harm or harm to others

• Severe or concerning side effects

• Dramatic changes in behavior or functioning

• Signs of allergic reaction

• Medical emergencies related to medication

WHEN TO CONTACT PARENTS:

• New or concerning side effects observed

• Changes in academic or social functioning

• Student reports feeling different or unwell

• Need to coordinate medication timing with home

GENERAL MONITORING TIPS:

√ Observe for 30 minutes after any new medication or dose change

√ Track patterns - when do side effects occur?

√ Note relationship between medication timing and symptoms

√ Document objectively, not subjectively

√ Coordinate observations with home and prescriber

√ Remember: most side effects are temporary and manageable

Emergency Contact: [Space for prescriber contact info]

School Protocol: [Space for school-specific procedures]

Developmental Considerations Table

MENTAL HEALTH BY DEVELOPMENTAL STAGE: QUICK REFERENCE

EARLY ELEMENTARY (AGES 5-7)

Normal Development:

• Concrete thinking, difficulty with abstract concepts

• Learning basic emotional vocabulary

• Beginning to understand rules and consequences

• Strong attachment to caregivers and teachers

• Play is primary way of processing experiences

Mental Health Presentations:

• Express distress through behavior and physical complaints

• Regression to earlier developmental stages when stressed

• Separation anxiety from caregivers

• Fears about safety of self and family

• Difficulty distinguishing reality from imagination

Assessment Considerations:

• Use simple, concrete language

• Observe behavior more than relying on verbal reports

327

- Include parent/teacher observations heavily

- Use play and art as assessment tools

- Focus on basic feelings (happy, sad, mad, scared)

Intervention Adaptations:

- Short attention span - brief interventions

- Use stories, games, and role-play

- Include parents/caregivers in treatment

- Focus on building emotional vocabulary

- Emphasize safety and predictability

LATE ELEMENTARY (AGES 8-11)

Normal Development:

- Developing logical thinking abilities

- Peer relationships becoming more important

- Beginning to understand others' perspectives

- Increased awareness of social rules and expectations

- Greater independence from parents

Mental Health Presentations:

- Can articulate feelings better but may still use physical complaints

- Academic performance anxiety becomes more common

- Peer rejection or bullying concerns

- Beginning awareness of being "different" from peers
- May try to hide problems to avoid being "bad"

Assessment Considerations:
- Can complete simple self-report measures with help
- Still benefit from behavioral observations
- Consider both home and school functioning
- Assess peer relationships and social skills
- Evaluate academic performance and school adjustment

Intervention Adaptations:
- Can engage in brief counseling sessions
- Benefit from skill-building approaches
- Group interventions can be effective
- Still need significant adult support and guidance
- Family involvement remains important

MIDDLE SCHOOL (AGES 12-14)

Normal Development:
- Abstract thinking abilities developing
- Identity formation begins
- Peer relationships central to self-esteem
- Physical changes of puberty

• Increased emotional intensity and mood swings

Mental Health Presentations:

• Depression and anxiety become more adult-like

• Self-harm behaviors may begin

• Eating disorder symptoms may emerge

• Social anxiety about peer acceptance

• Academic pressure and perfectionism

Assessment Considerations:

• Can complete standardized assessment tools

• Self-report becomes more reliable

• Consider peer relationships heavily

• Assess identity development and self-esteem

• Evaluate response to physical changes

Intervention Adaptations:

• Can engage in individual therapy

• Group interventions very effective

• Need balance of support and independence

• Address identity and self-esteem issues

• Include but don't over-involve parents

HIGH SCHOOL (AGES 15-18)

Normal Development:

• Advanced abstract thinking and planning abilities

• Identity consolidation

• Increasing independence from parents

• Future orientation and planning

• Romantic relationships become important

Mental Health Presentations:

• Adult-like mental health disorders

• Substance use experimentation

• Suicidal thoughts and behaviors peak

• Academic and social pressure intensify

• Future-oriented anxiety about college and careers

Assessment Considerations:

• Can complete adult assessment tools

• Self-report is generally reliable

• Consider developmental tasks and pressures

• Assess substance use and risky behaviors

• Evaluate future planning and goals

Intervention Adaptations:

- Can engage in individual therapy independently

- Benefit from cognitive-behavioral approaches

- Need respect for increasing autonomy

- Address future planning and identity issues

- Balance family involvement with independence

TRANSITION AGE (AGES 18-21)

Normal Development:

- Legal adulthood with continued brain development

- Transition to post-secondary education or work

- Developing intimate relationships

- Financial and practical independence

- Identity consolidation in adult roles

Mental Health Presentations:

- Continuation or emergence of serious mental illness

- Adjustment disorders related to life transitions

- Substance abuse concerns

- Relationship and intimacy issues

- Career and academic pressure

Assessment Considerations:

- Full adult assessment approaches

- Consider transition stressors and supports

- Assess practical life skills and independence

- Evaluate substance use patterns

- Consider impact on academic/work functioning

Intervention Adaptations:

- Adult treatment approaches

- Focus on practical life skills

- Address transition planning and support

- Consider family involvement based on student preference

- Coordinate with post-secondary support services

CULTURAL CONSIDERATIONS ACROSS ALL AGES:

- Family structure and decision-making patterns

- Communication styles and emotional expression

- Religious or spiritual perspectives on mental health

- Economic factors affecting access to care

- Language preferences and cultural concepts of illness

- Immigration status and acculturation stress

RED FLAGS AT ANY AGE:

- Suicidal thoughts or behaviors

- Self-harm or aggressive behaviors

- Substance abuse

- Severe withdrawal or isolation

- Dramatic changes in functioning

- Psychotic symptoms

- Trauma-related symptoms

Cultural Considerations in Mental Health

CULTURAL COMPETENCY QUICK REFERENCE FOR SCHOOL MENTAL HEALTH

COMMUNICATION STYLES BY CULTURAL BACKGROUND

HIGH-CONTEXT CULTURES (Asian, Latino, African, Native American)

- Communication includes nonverbal cues, silence, and implied meaning

- Direct questioning may feel intrusive or disrespectful

- Family hierarchy and elder respect affect who speaks for child

- Shame and honor concepts influence willingness to discuss problems

- Prefer relationship-building before discussing problems

Adaptation strategies:

✓ Spend time building rapport before assessment

✓ Include family members in appropriate ways

✓ Use indirect questioning and observation

✓ Respect silence and give time for responses

✓ Understand that "yes" may mean understanding, not agreement

LOW-CONTEXT CULTURES (European American, German, Scandinavian)

• Direct, explicit communication preferred

• Individual autonomy and self-advocacy valued

• Problem-focused discussions acceptable early in relationship

• Time efficiency often valued

• Written communication and documentation expected

Adaptation strategies:

✓ Provide clear, direct information about services

✓ Respect individual student's autonomy when age-appropriate

✓ Use structured assessment tools

✓ Provide written summaries and recommendations

✓ Be efficient but thorough in communications

MENTAL HEALTH CONCEPTS BY CULTURAL BACKGROUND

WESTERN/BIOMEDICAL MODEL

- Mental illness viewed as medical condition

- Individual treatment and medication accepted

- Professional help-seeking generally accepted

- Psychological causes and treatments understood

- Privacy and confidentiality highly valued

TRADITIONAL/INDIGENOUS MODELS

- Mental distress may be viewed as spiritual or community problem

- Healing often involves family, community, or spiritual leaders

- Traditional healing practices may be preferred or combined with Western treatment

- Collective responsibility for wellness

- Storytelling, ceremony, and ritual important in healing

RELIGIOUS/SPIRITUAL MODELS

- Mental distress may be viewed as spiritual crisis or test

- Prayer, faith community support, and pastoral care important

- Some resistance to secular mental health treatment

- Importance of hope, meaning, and purpose in healing

- Integration of faith and mental health treatment often preferred

FAMILY DYNAMICS AND DECISION-MAKING

COLLECTIVIST CULTURES

- Extended family involved in decisions about child

- Parents may defer to grandparents or other elders

- Children expected to prioritize family needs over individual needs

- Family reputation and honor considerations in treatment decisions

- Shame and stigma may prevent help-seeking

Adaptation strategies:

✓ Identify key decision-makers in family

✓ Include appropriate family members in meetings

✓ Address family concerns about stigma

✓ Frame treatment as helping family, not just individual

✓ Respect family hierarchy and communication patterns

INDIVIDUALIST CULTURES

- Parents typically primary decision-makers

- Individual child's needs prioritized

- Professional recommendations generally accepted

- Less extended family involvement in decisions

- Privacy and individual rights emphasized

Adaptation strategies:

✓ Work directly with parents as primary decision-makers

✓ Respect individual student's developing autonomy

✓ Provide individual-focused treatment recommendations

✓ Maintain confidentiality as appropriate

✓ Support student's individual goals and preferences

LANGUAGE AND INTERPRETATION

WORKING WITH INTERPRETERS

✓ Use trained medical interpreters when possible

✓ Avoid using family members, especially children, as interpreters

✓ Speak directly to student/family, not to interpreter

✓ Use first person ("I feel sad" not "She says she feels sad")

✓ Pause frequently for interpretation

✓ Ask interpreter to use exact words, not summaries

CONCEPTS THAT MAY NOT TRANSLATE

• "Depression" - may need to describe as "deep sadness" or "loss of energy"

• "Anxiety" - may need to describe as "excessive worry" or "fear"

• "Self-care" - concept may not exist or may seem selfish

• "Boundaries" - may conflict with cultural values about family closeness

• "Individual therapy" - may seem isolating or inappropriate

IMMIGRATION AND ACCULTURATION STRESS

RECENT IMMIGRANTS

- Language barriers affecting school performance
- Cultural adjustment stress
- Possible trauma from immigration experience
- Economic stress and uncertainty
- Loss of social status or professional identity

SECOND/THIRD GENERATION

- Cultural identity conflicts between home and school
- Pressure to succeed and represent family well
- Language switching between home and school
- Conflicting values about independence vs. family loyalty

REFUGEES AND ASYLUM SEEKERS

- Possible trauma from country of origin
- Ongoing uncertainty about legal status
- Grief and loss related to separation from homeland
- Survivor guilt about family members left behind
- Mistrust of authority figures including school staff

RELIGIOUS CONSIDERATIONS

INCORPORATING SPIRITUAL RESOURCES

√ Ask about religious or spiritual beliefs that provide comfort

√ Respect religious practices that support mental health

√ Coordinate with pastoral care when appropriate

√ Understand religious holidays and practices that affect school attendance

√ Address conflicts between religious beliefs and mental health treatment

POTENTIAL CONFLICTS

• Some religious beliefs may conflict with mental health treatment

• Stigma about mental illness in some religious communities

• Preference for prayer/faith over professional treatment

• Concerns about secular influences on children

GENDER ROLES AND EXPECTATIONS

TRADITIONAL GENDER ROLES

• Different expectations for boys vs. girls seeking help

• Some cultures discourage boys from expressing emotional distress

• Girls may have restrictions on interactions with male staff

• Family decision-making may be gender-based

LGBTQ+ CONSIDERATIONS

• Some cultures have strong prohibitions against non-heterosexual identities

• Family rejection or violence may be concerns

• Religious conflicts with LGBTQ+ identity

• Need for affirming support and possibly family mediation

PRACTICAL ADAPTATIONS

ASSESSMENT MODIFICATIONS

✓ Use culturally adapted assessment tools when available

✓ Include cultural stressors in assessment

✓ Consider cultural expressions of distress

✓ Ask about traditional healing practices

✓ Assess acculturation level and cultural identity

INTERVENTION MODIFICATIONS

✓ Include family as appropriate to culture

✓ Integrate cultural strengths and resources

✓ Address cultural stressors and discrimination

✓ Coordinate with cultural/religious leaders when appropriate

✓ Respect cultural healing practices

341

WORKING WITH CULTURAL LIAISONS

✓ Identify community cultural leaders and resources

✓ Build relationships with cultural organizations

✓ Attend cultural competency training regularly

✓ Consult with cultural experts on difficult cases

✓ Advocate for culturally responsive school policies

Remember: Culture is complex and individual - avoid stereotypes while being culturally responsive.

Technology and Social Media Impact Guide

TECHNOLOGY AND SOCIAL MEDIA IMPACT ON STUDENT MENTAL HEALTH

DEVELOPMENTAL DIFFERENCES IN TECHNOLOGY USE

ELEMENTARY (AGES 5-11)

Typical Use:

• Educational games and apps

• Limited social media (YouTube Kids, messaging with family)

• Beginning exposure to online content

• Screen time often supervised by adults

Mental Health Impacts:

• Sleep disruption from screen time before bed

• Attention difficulties from rapid content switching

• Early exposure to inappropriate content

• Comparison with unrealistic online images

• Cyberbullying beginning on gaming platforms

Warning Signs:

✓ Tantrums when screen time ends

✓ Difficulty sleeping after screen use

✓ Repetition of inappropriate language or behavior from online content

✓ Anxiety when separated from devices

✓ Decline in real-world play and social interaction

MIDDLE SCHOOL (AGES 12-14)

Typical Use:

• Social media platforms (Instagram, Snapchat, TikTok)

• Online gaming with strangers

• Text messaging and group chats

• Increased independence in online activities

Mental Health Impacts:

- Cyberbullying peaks during these years
- Social comparison and body image issues
- Fear of missing out (FOMO) from social media
- Sleep disruption from late-night device use
- Academic distraction from notifications and social drama

Warning Signs:

✓ Dramatic mood changes after device use

✓ Withdrawal from family and real-world friends

✓ Secretive behavior about online activities

✓ Sleep problems or fatigue at school

✓ Declining academic performance

✓ Anxiety when unable to check devices

✓ Body image concerns or diet changes

HIGH SCHOOL (AGES 15-18)

Typical Use:

- Multiple social media platforms simultaneously
- Dating apps and online relationships
- Academic pressure from online college information
- Job searching and professional networking beginning
- Increased exposure to news and world events online

Mental Health Impacts:

• Increased depression and anxiety linked to social media use

• Academic and social pressure from online comparison

• Exposure to harmful content (self-harm, eating disorders, substance use)

• Online drama affecting real-world relationships

• College and career pressure intensified by online information

Warning Signs:

√ Severe mood changes related to online interactions

√ Self-harm content in browsing history or social media

√ Dramatic changes in eating or exercise patterns

√ Social isolation in favor of online relationships

√ Academic decline due to technology distraction

√ Substance use content or behaviors influenced by online exposure

POSITIVE USES OF TECHNOLOGY FOR MENTAL HEALTH

BENEFICIAL APPLICATIONS:

√ Mental health apps for mood tracking and coping skills

√ Online therapy platforms for access to care

√ Educational content about mental health and wellness

✓ Support groups and communities for specific mental health concerns

✓ Crisis text lines and online support resources

✓ Mindfulness and meditation apps

RED FLAGS FOR HARMFUL TECHNOLOGY USE:

• Self-harm or suicide content creation or consumption

• Pro-eating disorder content engagement

• Online predators or inappropriate adult contact

• Cyberbullying as victim or perpetrator

• Excessive gaming interfering with basic needs

• Substance use content influencing behavior

• Sharing personal information that increases safety risk

SOCIAL MEDIA PLATFORMS AND MENTAL HEALTH RISKS

INSTAGRAM/SNAPCHAT:

Primary Risks:

• Image-focused content increases body dissatisfaction

• "Stories" create pressure for constant content creation

• Direct messaging enables private bullying

• Filtered images create unrealistic beauty standards

TIKTOK:

Primary Risks:

• Algorithm can promote harmful content (self-harm, eating disorders)

• Viral challenges sometimes dangerous or inappropriate

• Rapid content switching may affect attention spans

• Comments sections can be sources of bullying

GAMING PLATFORMS:

Primary Risks:

• Exposure to adult strangers through voice and text chat

• Addictive qualities affecting sleep, academics, and social relationships

• Toxic gaming culture and harassment

• In-game purchases creating financial stress

CYBERBULLYING RECOGNITION AND RESPONSE

SIGNS A STUDENT IS BEING CYBERBULLIED:

✓ Sudden reluctance to use devices previously enjoyed

✓ Emotional distress after checking messages or social media

✓ Withdrawal from social activities and friends

✓ Declining academic performance

√ Sleep disturbances or appetite changes

√ Reluctance to go to school or participate in activities

SIGNS A STUDENT IS CYBERBULLYING OTHERS:

√ Secretive behavior about online activities

√ Multiple accounts or fake profiles

√ Aggressive behavior that increases after device use

√ Lack of empathy about others' online experiences

√ Getting upset when device access is restricted

SCHOOL-BASED INTERVENTIONS:

√ Document cyberbullying incidents thoroughly

√ Coordinate with families of both victims and perpetrators

√ Involve law enforcement when threats or illegal behavior occur

√ Provide support for victims and consequences for perpetrators

√ Educate all students about digital citizenship

HEALTHY TECHNOLOGY USE GUIDELINES

RECOMMENDATIONS FOR FAMILIES:

√ Create device-free zones (bedrooms, dining areas)

√ Establish technology curfews before bedtime

✓ Model healthy technology use as adults

✓ Regularly review social media accounts and friend lists

✓ Educate about privacy settings and digital footprints

✓ Encourage face-to-face social interactions

SCHOOL STRATEGIES:

✓ Integrate digital citizenship education into curriculum

✓ Provide alternative activities that don't involve technology

✓ Create policies about device use during school hours

✓ Train staff to recognize technology-related mental health issues

✓ Partner with families on consistent technology expectations

CRISIS INTERVENTION FOR TECHNOLOGY-RELATED ISSUES:

✓ Take screenshots of concerning content before it's deleted

✓ Involve parents immediately for safety planning

✓ Report illegal content or behavior to appropriate authorities

✓ Provide mental health support for victims of online abuse

✓ Coordinate with social media platforms to remove harmful content

WHEN TO BE MOST CONCERNED:

• Student viewing or creating self-harm content

• Evidence of online predators or inappropriate adult contact

• Severe cyberbullying affecting daily functioning

• Gaming or social media use replacing sleep, eating, or school attendance

• Online activities supporting dangerous behaviors (substance use, risky challenges)

• Dramatic personality changes that coincide with new online activities

RESOURCES FOR FAMILIES:

✓ Common Sense Media for age-appropriate technology guidance

✓ ConnectSafely.org for digital safety information

✓ Local police departments for cyberbullying and online safety

✓ Mental health professionals with expertise in technology issues

✓ School counselors for digital citizenship education

Remember: Technology itself isn't harmful - it's how it's used that affects mental health. Focus on teaching healthy digital habits rather than avoiding technology entirely.

Warning Signs by Age Poster

MENTAL HEALTH WARNING SIGNS BY AGE

🔔 CALL FOR IMMEDIATE HELP:

• Threats of suicide or self-harm

- Aggressive behavior toward others

- Severe confusion or loss of touch with reality

- Substance use emergency

ELEMENTARY SCHOOL (AGES 5-11)

BEHAVIORAL CHANGES:

⚠ Sudden changes in eating or sleeping

⚠ Return to younger behaviors (thumb sucking, bed wetting)

⚠ Extreme clinginess or separation fears

⚠ Aggressive behavior or frequent tantrums

⚠ Social withdrawal from friends and activities

ACADEMIC/SOCIAL CHANGES:

⚠ Sudden drop in grades or school performance

⚠ Loss of interest in play or activities they used to enjoy

⚠ Complaints from teachers about behavior or attention

⚠ Frequent conflicts with peers

⚠ Reluctance to go to school

PHYSICAL/EMOTIONAL SIGNS:

⚠ Frequent complaints of headaches or stomachaches

⚠ Excessive worry about family members' safety

⚠ Persistent sadness or crying

⚠ Extreme fears that interfere with daily activities

⚠ Self-harm behaviors (hitting self, pulling hair)

MIDDLE SCHOOL (AGES 12-14)

MOOD/BEHAVIORAL CHANGES:

⚠ Extreme mood swings or irritability

⚠ Social withdrawal from family and friends

⚠ Loss of interest in activities and hobbies

⚠ Changes in friend groups or social circles

⚠ Risk-taking behaviors or rule-breaking

ACADEMIC/SOCIAL CHANGES:

⚠ Significant decline in academic performance

⚠ Skipping classes or school avoidance

⚠ Conflicts with teachers or authority figures

⚠ Bullying others or being bullied

⚠ Social media drama affecting daily life

PHYSICAL/EMOTIONAL SIGNS:

⚠ Changes in eating patterns or body image concerns

⚠ Sleep problems (too much or too little)

⚠ Self-harm behaviors (cutting, burning)

⚠ Excessive worry about appearance or peer acceptance

⚠ Panic attacks or severe anxiety episodes

HIGH SCHOOL (AGES 15-18)

MOOD/BEHAVIORAL CHANGES:

⚠ Persistent sadness, hopelessness, or emptiness

⚠ Extreme mood swings or emotional instability

⚠ Increased substance use or experimentation

⚠ Reckless or dangerous behavior

⚠ Giving away possessions or making final arrangements

ACADEMIC/SOCIAL CHANGES:

⚠ Dramatic drop in grades or school performance

⚠ Chronic absenteeism or truancy

⚠ Loss of motivation for future goals

⚠ Isolation from friends and family

⚠ Conflicts in romantic relationships

PHYSICAL/EMOTIONAL SIGNS:

⚠ Significant weight loss or gain

⚠ Changes in personal hygiene or appearance

⚠ Fatigue or loss of energy

⚠ Self-harm behaviors or suicide attempts

⚠ Expressions of worthlessness or guilt

WHEN MULTIPLE WARNING SIGNS ARE PRESENT:

✓ Duration: Signs persist for 2+ weeks

✓ Intensity: Signs interfere with daily functioning

✓ Change: Represents significant change from usual behavior

✓ Multiple areas: Affects home, school, and social functioning

IMMEDIATE ACTION STEPS:

1. Ensure student safety

2. Don't leave student alone if safety concerns exist

3. Contact parents/guardians

4. Document observations and actions taken

5. Refer for professional mental health evaluation

6. Follow school crisis protocols

SUPPORTIVE RESPONSES:

✓ "I've noticed some changes and I'm concerned about you"

✓ "Thank you for trusting me with this information"

✓ "You're not alone - there are people who want to help"

✓ "Let's figure out some ways to help you feel better"

AVOID SAYING:

✗ "Everyone goes through this"

✗ "Just think positive"

✗ "You have so much to live for"

✗ "This is just a phase"

✗ "Other kids have it worse"

Appendix D: Professional Resources

National Crisis Hotlines and Text Lines

CRISIS RESOURCES FOR STUDENTS AND FAMILIES

24/7 NATIONAL HOTLINES:

988 Suicide & Crisis Lifeline

• Available 24/7/365 for anyone in suicidal crisis or emotional distress

• Trained counselors provide support and local resource connections

• Available in English and Spanish

• Chat option available at suicidepreventionlifeline.org

• Serves all ages - children, teens, and adults

Crisis Text Line

• Text HOME to 741741

• Free, confidential, 24/7 crisis intervention via text

• Trained crisis counselors respond typically within 5 minutes

• Serves all ages

• Also available via WhatsApp and Facebook Messenger

National Child Abuse Hotline

- 1-800-4-A-CHILD (1-800-422-4453)

- 24/7 hotline for reporting child abuse and connecting families with local resources

- Available in 170+ languages

- Professional counselors and social workers staff the line

SPECIALIZED CRISIS LINES:

LGBTQ+ Resources:

The Trevor Project - 1-866-488-7386

- Crisis intervention and suicide prevention for LGBTQ+ youth under 25

- Available 24/7/365

- Also offers text (678678) and chat support

- TrevorLifeline.org

Trans Lifeline - 877-565-8860

- Peer support hotline run by trans people for trans and questioning individuals

- Not a crisis hotline but provides support and resources

PFLAG National Hotline - 1-202-467-8180

- Support for families and friends of LGBTQ+ individuals

Substance Abuse:

SAMHSA National Helpline - 1-800-662-4357

• Free, confidential, 24/7 treatment referral service

• Information about local treatment facilities, support groups, and community organizations

• Available in English and Spanish

Eating Disorders:

National Eating Disorders Association (NEDA) - 1-800-931-2237

• Information, support, and referrals for eating disorders

• Chat and text options available

• Screening tools available online

Domestic Violence:

National Domestic Violence Hotline - 1-800-799-7233

• 24/7 support for anyone experiencing domestic violence

• Available in 200+ languages

• Chat option available at thehotline.org

CRISIS TEXT LINES FOR SPECIFIC POPULATIONS:

Crisis Text Line Keywords:

• Text HOME to 741741 (general crisis support)

• Text HELLO to 741741 (for anxiety, depression, or emotional distress)

• Text LOVEIS to 22522 (for dating violence)

INTERNATIONAL STUDENTS:

International Association for Suicide Prevention

• Maintains list of crisis centers worldwide

• iasp.info/resources/Crisis_Centres/

LOCAL RESOURCES TO IDENTIFY:

✓ Local crisis hotlines and mobile crisis teams

✓ Emergency departments with psychiatric services

✓ Community mental health crisis services

✓ Local police crisis intervention teams

✓ Cultural and language-specific crisis resources

RESOURCES FOR SCHOOL STAFF:

Employee Assistance Programs (EAP)

• Many school districts offer confidential counseling for staff

• Check with HR about available services

Mental Health First Aid

- Training program for recognizing signs of mental health crises
- mentalhealthfirstaid.org

Crisis Prevention Institute (CPI)

- Training in de-escalation and crisis intervention
- crisisprevention.com

MOBILE APPS FOR CRISIS SUPPORT:

MY3 - Support Network

- Create personalized safety plan with 3 support contacts
- Includes warning signs, coping strategies, and crisis resources

notOK App

- One-touch button to alert trusted contacts during crisis
- Sends GPS location and pre-written message

Crisis Text Line for Schools

- Schools can text SCHOOL to 741741 for crisis support resources
- Provides guidance for school personnel dealing with student crises

WHEN TO USE DIFFERENT RESOURCES:

988 Suicide & Crisis Lifeline:

• Any mention of suicide or self-harm

• Severe depression or hopelessness

• Family member concerned about loved one's safety

• Need for immediate crisis intervention

Crisis Text Line:

• Students who prefer texting over talking

• Situations where phone calls aren't private

• Anxiety or panic attacks

• Emotional support during difficult times

Specialized Hotlines:

• Population-specific concerns (LGBTQ+, substance use, etc.)

• Need for specialized expertise

• Cultural or language-specific support needs

Local Crisis Services:

• Need for in-person evaluation or intervention

• Mobile crisis team response

• Follow-up after initial crisis contact

TRAINING CRISIS RESOURCES:

For School Staff:

✓ Mental Health First Aid for Schools

✓ Question, Persuade, Refer (QPR) suicide prevention training

✓ Applied Suicide Intervention Skills Training (ASIST)

✓ Crisis Prevention Institute (CPI) training

✓ Psychological First Aid

For Students:

✓ Peer support training programs

✓ Mental health awareness presentations

✓ Suicide prevention education programs

✓ Social-emotional learning curricula with crisis recognition

Remember: Always have multiple crisis resources available and ensure students know how to access help both during and after school hours.

Professional Development Opportunities

PROFESSIONAL DEVELOPMENT FOR SCHOOL NURSES IN MENTAL HEALTH

CERTIFICATION PROGRAMS:

National Board for Certification of School Nurses (NBCSN)

• Certified School Nurse (CSN) credential

• Includes mental health competencies

• Continuing education requirements maintain certification

• nationalbrdcertifiedschoolnurses.org

Mental Health First Aid

• 8-hour certification course

• Learn to identify, understand, and respond to signs of mental health crises

• Youth Mental Health First Aid specifically for ages 12-18

• mentalhealthfirstaid.org

• Available in-person and online formats

Crisis Prevention Institute (CPI)

• Nonviolent Crisis Intervention certification

• De-escalation and safe physical intervention techniques

• 6-hour initial training with annual recertification

• crisisprevention.com

SPECIALIZED TRAINING PROGRAMS:

Suicide Prevention:

QPR (Question, Persuade, Refer)

- 1-3 hour training program

- Teaches how to recognize suicide warning signs

- Available online and in-person

- qprinstitute.com

Applied Suicide Intervention Skills Training (ASIST)

- Intensive 2-day workshop

- Learn to provide immediate intervention for someone at risk

- Hands-on practice with role-playing scenarios

- livingworks.net

safeTALK

- Half-day training program

- Prepares participants to identify and connect at-risk individuals with resources

- Often combined with ASIST training

Trauma-Informed Care:

National Child Traumatic Stress Network

- Free online learning modules

- Trauma-informed care for schools

- Secondary trauma prevention for staff

- nctsn.org

Psychological First Aid for Schools

• National Center for PTSD training

• Learn to provide immediate support after traumatic events

• Focus on school-specific applications

• ptsd.va.gov

CONTINUING EDUCATION OPPORTUNITIES:

National Association of School Nurses (NASN)

• Annual conference with mental health tracks

• Webinar series on current topics

• Position statements and practice guidelines

• Online continuing education modules

• nasn.org

American Academy of Pediatrics (AAP)

• School health courses including mental health components

• Mental Health Minute webinar series

• Policy statements on school mental health

• aap.org

National Association of Secondary School Principals (NASSP) •
Mental health resources for school leaders • Crisis response planning
materials • Professional development webinars • principals.org

American School Health Association (ASHA) • Annual conference with mental health sessions • Journal of School Health with research updates • Professional development opportunities • ashaweb.org

SPECIALIZED CERTIFICATIONS:

Certified School Mental Health Specialist • Offered through various universities • 15-30 credit hour programs • Focus on school-based mental health interventions • Check with local universities for availability

Trauma-Informed Care Certification • Various organizations offer certification • Focus on recognizing and responding to trauma in schools • Includes secondary trauma prevention for staff

RESEARCH AND EVIDENCE-BASED PRACTICES:

National Center for School Mental Health (NCSMH) • University of Maryland-based resource center • Research briefs and implementation guides • Quality assessment tools for school mental health programs • schoolmentalhealth.org

Center for School Mental Health Analysis and Action • UCLA-based center • Research on effective school mental health practices • Policy recommendations and implementation resources • smhcollaborative.org

FUNDING OPPORTUNITIES:

Grant Programs to Research: • SAMHSA mental health promotion grants • CDC injury and violence prevention grants • Department of Education safe schools grants • Local foundation grants for school mental health • State-specific mental health funding opportunities

Professional Organization Scholarships: • NASN Foundation scholarships for continuing education • State nursing organization educational grants • Local healthcare foundation professional development funds

NETWORKING OPPORTUNITIES:

366

Professional Organizations to Join: • National Association of School Nurses (NASN) • State school nurse associations • American School Health Association • National Association of School-Based Health Centers

Online Communities: • NASN member forums • LinkedIn school health professional groups • Facebook groups for school nurses • State-specific school health networks

STAYING CURRENT WITH RESEARCH:

Key Journals to Follow: • Journal of School Health • The Journal of School Nursing • School Mental Health journal • Journal of School Violence • Pediatrics (American Academy of Pediatrics)

Research Databases: • PubMed for medical research • ERIC for educational research • PsycINFO for psychology research • Google Scholar for interdisciplinary research

Professional Development Planning:

1. **Assess current competencies** against professional standards

2. **Identify gaps** in knowledge or skills

3. **Set learning goals** for professional growth

4. **Create timeline** for completing training

5. **Seek funding** through employers or professional organizations

6. **Document learning** for certification maintenance

7. **Apply knowledge** in practice settings

8. **Evaluate impact** on student outcomes

Appendix E: Digital Resources

Mobile App Recommendations

FOR SCHOOL NURSES:

CrisisGo • Emergency communication and response platform • Coordinates with local emergency services • Real-time incident reporting and management

Epocrates • Drug reference guide including psychiatric medications • Drug interaction checker • Dosing calculator and side effect information

Mental Health Screening Apps: • ASQ Toolkit App (when available) • PHQ-9 Mobile • GAD-7 Screening Tool

FOR STUDENTS:

Crisis Support Apps: • MY3 - Personal safety planning • notOK - One-touch crisis alert system • Crisis Text Line - Direct access to crisis counselors

Mental Health Management: • Headspace - Meditation and mindfulness • Calm - Sleep stories and anxiety management • Sanvello - Anxiety and depression tracking • MindShift - CBT-based anxiety management

FOR FAMILIES:

Parent Resources: • Circle Home Plus - Screen time and content management • Qustodio - Digital wellness for families • Mental Health America Apps - Educational resources • NAMI - Local support group finder

Online Assessment Platforms

School-Based Platforms:

Panorama Education • Social-emotional learning surveys • Climate and culture assessments • Integration with school information systems • panoramaed.com

SAEBRS (Social, Academic, and Emotional Behavior Risk Screener) • Universal screening for behavioral risk • Progress monitoring capabilities • Research-based cut scores for decision making

FastBridge • Academic and behavior screening • Progress monitoring tools • Data management and reporting • fastbridge.org

Security and Privacy Considerations: • FERPA-compliant data storage • Encryption of sensitive information • User access controls and audit trails • Regular security updates and monitoring

Telehealth Resource Guides

Platforms for Student Mental Health:

Hazel Health • School-based telehealth services • Mental health counseling and support • Integration with school health programs • hazelhealth.com

TimelyCare • 24/7 mental health support for students • Crisis intervention capabilities • Counseling and psychiatric services • timelycare.com

Rula • Network of mental health providers • Insurance coverage verification • Appointment scheduling and management • rula.com

Implementation Considerations: • Technology requirements and compatibility • Staff training on platform use • Student and family orientation • Privacy and confidentiality protocols • Integration with existing school systems

Quality Assurance: • Licensed provider verification • Clinical supervision requirements • Outcome measurement and reporting • Regular platform evaluation and updates

Appendix F: Emergency Procedures

One-Page Crisis Protocols

SUICIDE RISK PROTOCOL

IMMEDIATE ACTIONS (First 5 Minutes):

1. Stay calm and ensure student safety

2. Do NOT leave student alone

3. Remove any means of harm from immediate area

4. Use ASQ screening questions if not already completed

5. Document exact words and behaviors

RISK ASSESSMENT: • Low Risk: Thoughts without plan or means • Moderate Risk: Thoughts with some planning • High Risk: Plan, means, and intent present

REQUIRED NOTIFICATIONS: • Parents/Guardians: Immediate contact required • Administration: Notify principal or designee • Crisis Team: Activate if available • Emergency Services: If imminent danger present

SAFETY PLANNING: • Identify warning signs with student • Develop coping strategies for school hours • Identify safe people and safe spaces • Create follow-up schedule • Coordinate with outside providers

DOCUMENTATION REQUIRED: • Time and location of incident • Exact statements made by student • Risk level assessment and rationale • All people notified and when • Safety measures implemented • Follow-up plans established

SELF-HARM PROTOCOL

IMMEDIATE MEDICAL ASSESSMENT:

1. Evaluate severity of injuries

2. Provide necessary first aid

3. Document injuries with photos if appropriate

4. Determine if emergency medical care needed

5. Contact parents about medical status

SAFETY CONSIDERATIONS: • Remove or secure potential self-harm tools • Implement continuous supervision • Assess ongoing risk for self-harm • Develop safety plan for school environment • Coordinate with mental health providers

REQUIRED ACTIONS: • Medical treatment of injuries • Parent notification about incident • Mental health evaluation referral • Safety planning and monitoring • Follow-up with outside providers

AGGRESSIVE BEHAVIOR PROTOCOL

IMMEDIATE SAFETY MEASURES:

1. Ensure safety of all students and staff

2. Remove other students from immediate area

3. Call for backup support if needed

4. Use de-escalation techniques

5. Document incident thoroughly

DE-ESCALATION STRATEGIES: • Remain calm and speak slowly • Give student physical space • Use non-threatening body language • Validate feelings while setting boundaries • Offer choices when possible

POST-INCIDENT PROCEDURES: • Medical assessment for injuries • Support for all affected students • Parent notification and meeting • Behavioral intervention planning • Coordination with administration

Emergency Contact Sheets

INTERNAL SCHOOL CONTACTS

Principal: [Name, Phone, Email] **Assistant Principal:** [Name, Phone, Email] **School Counselor:** [Name, Phone, Email] **School Psychologist:** [Name, Phone, Email] **Security/Resource Officer:** [Name, Phone, Email] **District Crisis Team:** [Phone, Pager] **Superintendent's Office:** [Phone, After-hours contact]

EXTERNAL EMERGENCY SERVICES

911 Emergency Services Local Police Department: [Non-emergency number] **Fire Department:** [Non-emergency number] **Emergency Medical Services:** [Direct contact if available]

MENTAL HEALTH CRISIS SERVICES

988 Suicide & Crisis Lifeline Crisis Text Line: Text HOME to 741741 **Local Mobile Crisis Team:** [Phone, Coverage hours] **Local Crisis Center:** [Phone, Address] **Emergency Department with Psych Services:** [Hospital name, Phone]

CHILD PROTECTIVE SERVICES

State CPS Hotline: [24-hour number] **Local CPS Office:** [Phone, After-hours contact] **CPS Investigation Unit:** [Direct contact if available]

SPECIALIZED CRISIS SERVICES

Poison Control: 1-800-222-1222 **Domestic Violence Hotline:** 1-800-799-7233 **Child Abuse Hotline:** 1-800-422-4453 **Substance Abuse Crisis Line:** [Local contact]

Incident Command System Integration

SCHOOL CRISIS RESPONSE ROLES

Incident Commander (Usually Principal): • Overall response coordination • Resource allocation decisions • Media and external communication • Parent and family communication coordination

Operations Chief (Usually Assistant Principal): • Student and staff accounting • Evacuation and shelter procedures • Security and crowd control • Emergency services coordination

Planning Chief (Usually Counselor/Nurse): • Crisis response plan implementation • Resource needs assessment • Documentation coordination • Recovery planning

Logistics Chief (Usually School Secretary/Manager): • Communication systems management • Supply and equipment coordination • Transportation arrangements • Facility management

MENTAL HEALTH SPECIFIC ROLES

School Nurse: • Medical triage and treatment • Mental health crisis assessment • Coordination with emergency medical services • Family notification for medical issues

School Counselor/Psychologist: • Psychological first aid • Crisis counseling services • Trauma response coordination • Long-term mental health planning

Mental Health Crisis Team: • Severe mental health emergency response • Risk assessment and safety planning • Professional mental health evaluation • Hospitalization coordination if needed

COMMUNICATION PROTOCOLS

Internal Communication: • Regular check-ins every 15-30 minutes during active crisis • Use designated communication channels (radios, phones) • Document all major decisions and actions • Maintain chain of command

External Communication: • Single spokesperson designated (usually principal) • Prepared statements for media if needed • Regular updates to district office • Coordination with emergency services

Disaster Response Mental Health Procedures

IMMEDIATE RESPONSE (First 24 Hours)

Psychological First Aid Principles:

1. Promote safety and calm

2. Promote connectedness

3. Instill hope and efficacy

4. Promote collaborative services

5. Promote calm

Initial Mental Health Actions: • Assess immediate psychological casualties • Provide basic comfort and support • Connect people with social supports • Protect from additional harm • Provide information about normal stress reactions

HIGH-RISK POPULATIONS TO MONITOR: • Students with pre-existing mental health conditions • Students who witnessed traumatic events directly • Students with limited family support • Students with previous trauma history • Staff members affected by the disaster

SHORT-TERM RESPONSE (First Week)

Screening and Assessment: • Brief screening for all students and staff • More detailed assessment for high-risk individuals • Referral for professional evaluation when needed • Ongoing monitoring of adjustment

Support Services: • Group processing sessions for affected classes • Individual counseling for severely impacted students • Staff support and debriefing sessions • Family support and education

LONG-TERM RESPONSE (Weeks to Months)

Continued Monitoring: • Regular check-ins with identified at-risk students • Ongoing assessment of school climate and functioning • Monitoring for delayed stress reactions • Coordination with community mental health services

Recovery Planning: • Return to normal routines when appropriate • Memorial or acknowledgment activities if appropriate • Evaluation of crisis response effectiveness • Planning improvements for future events

Lockdown Mental Health Considerations

DURING LOCKDOWN PROCEDURES

Mental Health Priorities: • Remain calm and reassure students • Provide age-appropriate information • Model coping behaviors • Monitor for panic responses • Support students with special needs

Managing Student Anxiety: • Use quiet, reassuring voice tones • Teach simple breathing exercises • Redirect attention to calming activities • Maintain physical comfort when possible • Be honest but age-appropriate about situation

Supporting Students with Mental Health Conditions: • Identify students who may need extra support • Implement individual coping strategies • Monitor for increased anxiety or panic • Provide additional reassurance and support • Consider medication needs for long lockdowns

AFTER LOCKDOWN PROCEDURES

Immediate Debriefing: • Allow students to express feelings and concerns • Provide factual information about what happened • Normalize emotional reactions to the event • Identify students who need additional support • Connect students with families quickly when safe

Follow-Up Mental Health Support: • Screen all students for trauma reactions • Provide group processing opportunities • Offer individual counseling for affected students • Monitor for changes in behavior or academic performance • Coordinate with families about home support

Long-Term Considerations: • Continue monitoring affected students • Provide ongoing mental health services as needed • Review and improve lockdown mental health procedures • Train staff in trauma-informed responses • Build resilience and recovery into school culture

Your Complete Mental Health Toolkit

These appendices provide you with the practical tools, resources, and protocols you need to implement comprehensive mental health support in your school setting. From printable assessment forms to emergency procedures, these resources transform the knowledge you've gained throughout this handbook into actionable, ready-to-use materials.

The true value of these appendices lies not just in having good resources, but in knowing how to use them systematically and effectively. Regular practice with assessment tools, familiarity with crisis protocols, and ongoing professional development ensure that you're prepared to provide the highest quality mental health support for your students.

Your role as a school nurse places you at the center of student mental health support. These tools give you the confidence and competence to serve in that role while maintaining appropriate professional boundaries and legal compliance. The investment you make in organizing, practicing, and maintaining these resources pays dividends every time a student needs help and you're prepared to provide it.

Reference

American Academy of Child and Adolescent Psychiatry. (2018). *Patient Health Questionnaire-9 (PHQ-9) for adolescents.*

American Academy of Pediatrics. (2019). *HIPAA and FERPA basics.*

American Academy of Pediatrics. (2024). *HIPAA and FERPA basics.*

American School Counselor Association. (2024). *ASCA ethical standards for school counselors.*

California School-Based Health Alliance. (2024). *Comparing HIPAA and FERPA.*

California School-Based Health Alliance. (2024). *HIPAA FERPA guide – Key points about HIPAA and FERPA in California.*

California School-Based Health Alliance. (2024). *Student consent including mental health and sexual and reproductive health services.*

Centers for Disease Control and Prevention. (2024). *Facts about suicide.*

Centers for Disease Control and Prevention. (2024). *Health disparities in suicide prevention.*

Centers for Disease Control and Prevention. (2024). *Mental health and suicide risk among high school students – Youth Risk Behavior Survey, United States, 2023. MMWR Surveillance Summaries, 73(4), 1–15.*

Centers for Disease Control and Prevention. (2024). *Suicide facts and statistics.*

Centers for Disease Control and Prevention. (2024). *Youth Risk Behavior Survey data summary and trends report, 2013–2023.*

Columbia Lighthouse Project. (2024). *Columbia-Suicide Severity Rating Scale (C-SSRS) frequently asked questions.*

Columbia University Department of Psychiatry. (2024). *Columbia-Suicide Severity Rating Scale (C-SSRS).*

Defuse De-Escalation Training. (2024). *3 de-escalation techniques essential for mental health professionals.*

ERIC. (2019). *School reintegration post-psychiatric hospitalization: Protocols and procedures across the nation. School Mental Health, 11(3).*

Frontiers in Psychiatry. (2020). *Codesigning a mental health discharge and transitions of care intervention: A modified nominal group technique.*

Mandated Reporter Training. (2024). *What are nurses responsible for reporting?*

National Association of School Nurses. (2022). *Survey finds 45% of school nurses report mental health as top concern.*

National HIV Curriculum. (2024). *Generalized Anxiety Disorder 7-item (GAD-7) screening tool.*

National HIV Curriculum. (2024). *Patient Health Questionnaire-9 (PHQ-9) administration guide.*

National Institute of Mental Health. (2024). *Ask Suicide-Screening Questions (ASQ) toolkit materials.*

National Institute of Mental Health. (2024). *ASQ screening tool administration guide.*

NAMI Wisconsin. (2024). *Academic accommodations for students with mental health conditions.*

NCBI Bookshelf. (2024). *Chapter 2 therapeutic communication and the nurse-client relationship – Nursing: Mental health and community concepts.*

NCBI Bookshelf. (2024). *Mandatory reporting laws. StatPearls Publishing.*

Pennsylvania Department of Health. (2024). *Confidentiality/HIPAA/FERPA guidance for school health programs.*

PubMed Central. (2023). *The impact of social media on the mental health of adolescents and young adults: A systematic review.*

SchoolHouse Connection. (2024). *State laws on minor consent for routine medical care.*

Smith, J., Johnson, A., & Williams, K. (2024). Perfect storm: Emotionally based school avoidance in the post-COVID-19 pandemic context. *Journal of School Psychology, 102,* 234–251.

Soliant Health. (2024). *Open communication is a top tool for school nurses.*

Springer. (2019). *School reintegration post-psychiatric hospitalization: Protocols and procedures across the nation. School Mental Health, 11(3),* 495–508.

Substance Abuse and Mental Health Services Administration. (2024). *Behavioral health resources for youth in schools.*

Thomas, C. S., Nielsen, T. K., & Best, N. C. (2025). A rapid review of mental health training programs for school nurses. *The Journal of School Nursing, 41(1),* 23–35.

U.S. Department of Health and Human Services. (2023). *Social media and youth mental health: The U.S. Surgeon General's advisory 2023.*

Wisconsin Department of Children and Families. (2024). *Mandated child abuse and neglect reporters.*

Zero Suicide Institute. (2024). *Ask Suicide-Screening Questions (ASQ) toolkit implementation guide.*

www.ingramcontent.com/pod-product-compliance
Lightning Source LLC
Chambersburg PA
CBHW050450270326
41927CB00009B/1674